COUNSELLING ADOLESCENTS IN SCHOOL

Counselling Adolescents in School

Anne Jones

Kogan Page

Much of this book is based on information included in *School Counselling in Practice* published by Ward Lock Educational Co Ltd in 1970. There has been extensive revision with additional material.

This edition first published in 1977
by Kogan Page Limited
116a Pentonville Road, London N1 9JN

Printed in Great Britain by Anchor Press Ltd
and bound by Wm Brendon & Son Ltd
both of Tiptree, Essex

ISBN 0 85038 132 0

Contents

Acknowledgements

I want to thank all those people who helped me in my work as a counsellor and in the writing of this book, in particular, the former head and deputy head of Mayfield School, Dame Margaret Miles and Miss Helen Whale; my fellow counsellor at Mayfield, Mrs Shirley Dunkley, and my casework supervisor, Miss Mary Kernick. I also want to thank my former colleagues at Thomas Calton School, and all those other friends and colleagues who have advised, supported, and stimulated me over the years. Last, and most important of all, my husband and children for their encouragement, understanding and love.

I must make it clear that the views expressed in this book are my own and not necessarily those of my education authority or any of the people I have worked with over the years.

Anne Jones

Introduction

This book was originally written as an account of an experiment in counselling adolescents in a secondary school between 1965-1971. That part of the text remains substantially as it was written, but it is important to realize that it relates to a specific period in time, when I was working as counsellor at Mayfield School. There are two completely new chapters. In chapter 11, 'The counsellor as educator', I seek to explore ways in which counselling can serve and enhance the educational process. To this I have added a brief practical account of my work as deputy head of Thomas Calton School, with the aim of demonstrating both the usefulness and the relevance of counselling skills to the organization and development of a school. In chapter 1 I use the insights I have gained as a counsellor to look at the question of whether or not schools are working on the issues which really help adolescents grow up. In particular I focus on the relationship between school, careers guidance, and employment. I remain as convinced as ever that there is a place for counsellors in our schools. My hope however is that this book will help any adult working with adolescents to do his job better.

For those astute readers who notice that I appear to change sex during the book with alarming rapidity, let me explain that when I talk about the work I did when I was a counsellor I use the feminine case. When I talk about counselling in general I use the masculine, partly to make the important point that counselling is *not* a female prerogative—no sex discrimination here!

Finally I must make it clear that where I have quoted from individual comments or cases, I have taken great care to change names and remove identifying details. I have also changed details of the problems, though not in a substantial way, for I wanted the problems to be real, not fantasies invented for effect.

Anne Jones

Chapter 1

Counselling and adolescence: what now?

When the school counselling movement began in Britain in 1965, it was difficult to foresee what effects it would have. Those of us involved in the movement were excited and confident that counselling would add a vitally needed element to the education of the adolescent. These were expansionist times; for a while it looked as if there would eventually be a counsellor appointed in every school. The principles and concepts of counselling were seized upon with alacrity by many adults working with young people—not just teachers, but also careers officers, youth workers and social workers. There must have been something in the timing of the 'discovery' of the body of knowledge which already existed about counselling which rang a bell with those adults who were seeking to help adolescents in the 60s. The mood then was complex—as indeed it still is. There was a general questioning of the established order, of authority, of moral and social values. There was a feeling among adults sympathetic to young people that adolescents were not given enough say in their own destiny; they were too often told what to do, expected to conform to the rules 'because I say so'. Adults did not always listen sufficiently to what young people were saying; adults often failed to recognize their 'cry for help'; when they did try to help they too often were over-directive, or offered the help on terms which were unacceptable to young people. In many ways, the situation does not seem to have changed very much!

What is sure is that in 1965, certain counselling concepts—in particular the idea of being 'non-directive', non-judgemental and non-authoritarian—fell like manna not only on the ears of the teaching profession, but also of other agencies dealing with young people. Counselling and all its concepts seemed to be the answer for many of the helping professions.

Unfortunately but perhaps inevitably this was *not* all for the best in the best of all possible worlds. Instead of the steady building up of a truly professional body of counsellors, suddenly everyone was trying his hand, sometimes with unfortunate results. The result of this phase was, in my view, a devaluing of the word 'counselling' which was, and still is, frequently abused and misused; a surfeit of non-directive, non-judgemental, non-authoritarian helpers; considerable role confusion and role diffusion, particularly among teachers and social workers; the emergence of a very confused adolescent group who found the adult world apparently leaning over backwards to please them and not impose on them. I discuss these particular questions in more detail in chapter 11.

The picture I have just painted is of course exaggerated. We all know adults who were totally untouched by this phase! But those adults who went through it have been grappling since then with the problem of learning how to use their authority as adults, in relationship to adolescents; we have learnt that it does not help young people to grow up if we renounce our own authority, wisdom, experience and judgement as adults. The skill we have to develop consists of using these qualities constructively, not destructively; for example in being sensitive without being sentimental, strong without being overpowering, flexible without being flaccid, loving without being over-involved, gentle without being soft, firm without being rigid, tolerant without being ridiculous. Swinging about on the see-saw of polarization really does not help; we somehow have to learn to manage and to use both 'ends' of ourselves at once if we are really to help at all. This is something young people often see more clearly than we do.

However, the fact that counselling concepts have often been misunderstood and counselling techniques used inappropriately does not mean that they should not be used at all. The conflicts of adolescence (like the conflicts of adulthood!) are still with us, and still offer one of the best opportunities for growth and development that a person ever has. In schools and in society generally we have still not learnt how best to help adolescents use this period of conflict as a basis for growth. In the light of our experiences in the last few years, this may be a good moment to look again at the basic principles of counselling. They are in my view as relevant now as they ever were; an understanding of these principles and some experience in the techniques of counselling are vital to anyone working with young people.

Counselling and pastoral care

Why is it that we still do not have a counsellor appointed to every secondary school? The need is as great as ever, greater in many ways, particularly in an era of inner-urban decline, economic stringency and unemployment. Numbers of children in distress are higher than ever. Rutter's social adjustment scale, used in an Inner London Borough in 1971, showed a deviance rate of 19.1% (21.6% for boys, 16.5% for girls).[1] Compare this with Clegg's 1968 rough estimate of 10-12%.[2] A single parent, unemployment, chronic ill health, overcrowded and inadequate housing, poverty, lack of care: so many of our inner-city pupils battle against these background odds (and survive remarkably well) that those of us who work in inner-city schools begin, alas, to take such handicaps as normal. Add to these social and economic factors the very bleak prospects for employment which face so many of our young people, and you may well wonder why a counsellor is still considered a luxury. On the vocational guidance side alone there is more than a full-time job for a counsellor in every secondary school. Even if personal counselling is still considered a frill for the few, vocational guidance is surely a necessity for all.

The reasons why there are no full-time counsellors in all our secondary schools are both positive and negative. The negative reasons are largely economic. There is still no full-scale backing from the Department of Education and Science for this idea. As long as head teachers have to 'give up' a teacher to provide a counsellor, the odds are going to be set against the counsellor. The counsellor and his responsibility allowance will have to be *extra* to the quota for them to be taken up in a big way. Second, the supply of properly selected and trained counsellors is still small, despite the proliferation of training courses over the years[3] and the efforts of such bodies as NICEC[4] which also publishes a very respectable journal of guidance and counselling.[5] It would still be a mistake for the wrong people to take up this kind of work.

On the positive side, one reason counsellors have not 'spread' more may relate to their effectiveness. I have always maintained that one of the counsellor's objectives should be to do himself out of a job! Overall the quality of 'pastoral care', of careers advice and of educational guidance has improved over the last ten years. There is a greater degree of sensitivity and system in these areas now than there was. Many trained counsellors are not working officially as counsellors. They have taken posts in the school hierarchy where they have an opportunity of working on the system as well as with individuals. We can make analogies with other developments which have both a specialist and a generalist phase, for example health education, remedial teaching, and careers education. Are these specialist subjects to be taught and contained within a department, or are they to be taught by everybody 'across the curriculum'? My own view is that in all these areas, including counselling, we still need both approaches. The specialists can help train the staff as a whole as well as doing their own specialist work.

It is a relief to note therefore that even though there may not be an official counsellor, there is in the vast majority of secondary schools a pastoral care system, which is indeed systematic, structured and organized; with points and posts of responsibility allocated to it; with specific tasks to do apart from the day-to-day care and discipline, such as smoothing the transition from primary to secondary school, providing guidance for subject choices, offering careers advice and preparing for the transition from school to work. Interviews with parents and pupils and contacts with other agencies are conducted with a degree of professional skill and properly recorded; advice is sought from other agencies at a preventive stage, and decisions about pupils' future welfare are properly communicated to the appropriate persons. Indeed in many schools the recording and assessing of social and psychological problems and behavioural difficulties may well be done more meticulously than the assessing of academic progress.

Why is it then that I am still not satisfied? I have already mentioned that there are some institutions and some people who remain untouched by the development of the last decade or so. I am concerned lest in the 'tightening up of standards' of work and behaviour which is with us now, we will lose the gains we have made. There still do exist some teachers who work in a way which is over-rigid and over-controlling. Their pupils either give up and are rejected out of hand, or they become conformist and over-dependent. Their problems come when they leave school and discover that they have been over-protected all their school lives. This extreme of teacher behaviour is just as unhelpful to the adolescent as that of the teacher who overindulges his pupils another way, by forgiving everything and forgetting to teach them to take responsibility for the consequences of their action. In spite of the counselling movement, both these extremes of teacher behaviour still exist and still need working on. Furthermore, the pastoral care system can be completely undermined if some staff are operating on a different wavelength from the school as a whole. The mechanisms of the system do not tell you much about the *nature* of the pastoral care. The system can be about the *control* of pupils or it can be about the *growth* of pupils. True education like true counselling is interested in growth from within, not control from without.

Further, it is a mistake for the pastoral care system to be *grafted* on to the academic system and split from it: more of this in chapter 11. Pupils' learning comes from their total experience of the school, not simply from what goes on in lessons. Some of the messages given out by schools are contradictory and *not* conducive to pupil growth and development. If the 'caring' and the 'learning' parts of the school experience are split, then the pupil may feel himself in a kind of fragmented chaos of which it is difficult to make any sense. Caring and learning need to be integrated; so do loving and making demands on pupils. Something radical has gone wrong here. Teachers are now making a real attempt, in response to popular demands, to achieve 'higher standards'. Yet so often this attempt comes across to the pupils as hysterical meaningless nagging, against which they are well defended. All that happens then is that a larger proportion of the pupil population than before becomes alienated from school. As teachers we have to learn how to convey that because we care about the pupils' progress as *pupils,* we are prepared to make demands on our pupils *and* give them the support and the skills they need to fulfil those demands. This does not demean the pupil. On the contrary, it is putting up with less than a pupil's best which is the real insult. Our job as teachers is to support and encourage the pupil in his battle to do his best and move forward, not to make it so easy for him that he does not bother any more. Teachers often appear to accept shoddy work because they are afraid of upsetting the pupil. Yet cushioning against reality does nothing to help the pupil. As teachers we have to learn how to convey a *total* message; we too often appear to be alternately overindulgent or over-rejecting, because the message is split into two parts. These principles, of being firm because we care, of accepting the pupil without either condoning or rejecting him, of making demands on the pupil so that *he* works it out for himself with our support, are principles which apply equally to teaching and to counselling. They are also principles which still continue to be misunderstood and misapplied, and need a lot of working on if schools are to be anything more than child-minding agencies. In some ways secondary schools seem to prolong childhood rather than promote adulthood.

Where does the form teacher stand now in all this? Often in danger of splitting himself into two separate people, the form teacher and the class teacher. It is clear that form teachers have a vitally important role, especially for pupils with deprived home circumstances. Yet the dangers for the conscientious form teacher have been in taking on too much and getting too involved. Teachers are not primarily social workers, friends or even parents to their pupils. How form teachers will understand and take up their role will depend on how well they are trained and co-ordinated in their school. I agree with Michael Marland's concept of the 'tutor ascendant'.[6] The more responsibility they are allowed to exercise, the more responsible they are likely to be. If they make mistakes, never mind, they will learn. We tend to protect both our teachers and our pupils from making mistakes and taking risks; yet this is a most valuable part of learning. Certainly most form teachers are willing and capable of taking on a considerable counselling role if given the support and the opportunity. I suspect that there is still much under-functioning here, largely because of confusion over role and over the delegation of responsibility. The more form teachers understand the true principles of counselling the better. One of those principles lies in the recognition of the boundaries and the limitations of roles.

Counselling and careers

The question of careers advice is one which is even more fraught with difficulties now than it was when the counselling movement began. Careers teachers had of course been established in schools long before then, but the concept of careers guidance, as opposed to advice, was one which developed as part of the counselling movement. 'Guidance programmes' sprang up over the country. Now we are into yet another phase—careers education.[7] In theory at least, the pupil has never been so well prepared for deciding what to do with his future. Normally from about the third year on he is given lessons, lectures and individual consultations designed to help him think about his own aptitudes, abilities and personality, his strengths and limitations; to help him choose the right options; to help him find out about as many jobs as possible and the life styles that go with them; to help him make a decision, with the help of the careers teacher and the careers officer, about what he wants to do.

Yet even thus far we find there are snags. First, some schools seem curiously reluctant to differentiate between pupils or to assess their ability objectively. The reluctance comes from a belief in the unreliability of testing procedures, and the negative effects of putting pupils in rank order for those who are not top. Both these points have some validity, yet the corollary, which is that because this is difficult to do well, nothing much is done at all, makes it very hard for a pupil to know how well he is getting on either in relationship to his own potential, or in relationship to his peers. There may well be more mute inglorious Miltons around then ever! If a pupil is to think about his abilities at all usefully, he needs to have more than his own thoughts to work with, however accurate they might happen to be. As far as options and job choices are concerned, the whole exercise may be very remote and second-hand for the pupil. Whose word is he to believe? Which PR film will take his fancy? And how much will the careers personnel really help him—or will he still prefer to believe what his peers and his parents say about jobs? And *is* it a final choice? Maybe it is just a first choice, and not really all that important.

There are other inherent difficulties in this new sophisticated stage of careers education. Parents and friends, subject teachers, heads of house, form tutors, careers teachers, counsellors, careers officers—all these people, for a start, may be involved in advising or guiding a pupil. What does the pupil make of it all? How consistent or how coherent is what he hears? A further complication, alas only too real, is that jobs for school leavers, with or without qualifications, are getting harder to find. This can unfortunately make careers advice seem like a 'con' designed in part to get better examination results for the school. The desperate exhortations of the teacher to make pupils work harder for qualifications may fall on very deaf ears when pupils know perfectly well that there are not any real prospects. There is no doubt that progress has been made in the field of careers education and guidance. There is a lot of hard work going on. But are we working on the right issues? In many ways we may still be missing the point.

In the teaching of reading there is a well worn concept called 'reading readiness'. I suspect that there may be a similar concept in careers guidance. At certain times pupils may be totally unreceptive to guidance because they are working on some other problem. This is not a chronological state so much as a developmental stage. For example, a pupil may not be ready to think about his future career in terms of what *he* really wants, because he is at the stage where his 'choice' is *reaction* against something rather than an action in its own right. He may want to leave school at 16 *because* his parents want him to stay on or vice versa. Can we or do we do anything about this?

Alternatively he may want to do something simply because he has not thought at all. Dad is a long-distance lorry-driver, so he (being masculine like dad) will naturally want to be a long-distance lorry-driver. So, as he does not need qualifications for this, school doesn't matter at all, thank you very much. What can we or should we do about this?

And what about the pupil who has unrealistic ambitions in spite of all our advice? It is a very long and subtle job helping a pupil work through this, especially when he is supported in his *idée fixe* by ambitious parents who can put intolerable pressure on their offspring. Very few of our existing mechanisms for careers guidance allow enough time to work on this. Should we do more about it?

More normally pupils, especially girls, will have unimaginative and depressed aspirations;[8] they will not take up the range of opportunities open to them even when they are told about them time and time again. They will be unwilling to take the risk of doing something unfamiliar, or to travel far to work, or to move home in order to train or have a better job. What is it that we are or are not doing in schools for this kind of attitude to prevail? Overcoming this kind of attitude takes much more than a few careers lessons. There are now available a few teaching materials which are aimed at these issues.[9] But attitudes here go deep. It is not so much a careers programme but more a way of life that we have to consider.

What schools often underestimate is how much school life contributes to attitudes as well as home life. Schools cannot do everything—but in rightly denying the charge that they can put the wrongs of society right, they sometimes make it sound as if they have *no* contribution at all to make to pupil attitudes. Seven hours a day, five days a week is a considerable amount of time. It is certainly more time than average working parents spend with their family, particularly if they are single parents. The question of the total message conveyed by a school is something of great significance. I shall return to this point later.

Much has been said and written over the years about the importance of preparing pupils for life, in particular the importance of 'good working habits' and equally 'learning to make decisions and choices for oneself'. I have a feeling that on both these scores, schools still have hardly begun. When the emphasis in lessons is on academic achievement then the pupil may learn to deliver the goods but not sufficiently develop his own resources. When the emphasis is on 'creativity' and 'individualized research methods' then the pupil may not learn to work in a team to some objective; that is to say, the pupil may have goals of his own (or he may not!) but he may fail to learn to value and respond to the setting of external objectives by his class or school, other than the purely selfish one of passing exams. This may say more about the way schools operate than about the individual child. I am making a rather subtle point which is to do with the overindulgence of the individual and his whims (which may be good, bad or indifferent) and the *lack* of what used to be called 'corporate goals'. This whole tendency is also often reflected in the staffs of schools who work splendidly in individualistic ways, but often in ways which do not fit together to make sense as a whole. At one end of the scale we have the battery-hen approach to education, turning out examination fodder (or examination rejects); at the other end of the scale, we have individuals who may be massively under achieving, but in any case who may not have learnt to use their talents in the service of the school. For school, read any institution in which they may later work.

In a work situation employers do *not* want battery hens—they want to harness and use the constructive energy of their staff. But neither do they want creative geniuses (or uncreative nuisances) who lack a sense of corporate identity and corporate achievement. So this is a big issue of which anyone in careers work needs to be aware. The 'careers programme' will be nothing unless the school as a whole and the staff as a whole are agreed on the importance of this in every aspect of school life. In a seven-hour school day, lessons will take up only four and a half hours or so. What does the pupil learn from the other two and a half hours in school? Who cares what goes on then? Whether he likes to face this or not, the teacher's job does not end when the lesson is finished. All the time he is in school he is, wittingly or not, conveying a message to the pupils. What kind of message will depend on the school and its corporate ethos. The pupil's basic attitude to adults, to employment, to the world of work and to his future role in society will be much influenced by whatever kind of 'school life' he experiences.[10] This point may seem remote from counselling and careers. It is not. It is part of my overall thesis that the effectiveness of the parts depends upon the functioning of the whole.

As for learning to make choices and decisions, this important area, in terms of helping adolescents become more effective adults, is still often practically untouched in schools. The question of 'subject options' may well be dealt with thoroughly but how much real choice is there, and who actually makes it? As a pupil once said, 'Is this a choice, Miss, or can we do what we like?' Like so many parts of schooling, learning to make choices is *not* a free for all subject. It requires system and planning and above all an understanding on the part of the pupil as to *why* he is being asked to do something. Again this is an idea which can be taken up mistakenly by the teacher, like the English class who were always given a choice of what *kind* of work they wanted to do in English, and nearly always chose 'creative writing'. The result was that they were not sufficiently exposed to other, equally important, kinds of experience in the English language. The skill is not in offering a choice between pease pudding and ice cream; it is perhaps in putting the question another way—making the pupil work out for himself that he does need to develop a certain skill or ability, and having him agree that to make the best of himself he needs to do certain specific learning tasks. If we simply give our pupils a choice between learning or not learning, their choice may be based on the wrong premise. If they understand *why* this piece of work may help them in their development as adults, then they are more likely to take it up. It helps if the teachers themselves believe the piece of work to be useful and they themselves know why it is useful—otherwise the teacher may be pushing into the pupil his own basic doubts about the validity of what he is doing. To my mind this kind of understanding of the purposes of education is essential if the secondary education system is to continue to meet the needs of our young people and our society at all.

So much for 'choice' and purpose within subject lessons. But what about the 'decision-making exercises' of which we all had such hope? Despite all the froth and ferment of ideas, there seems to be very little genuine participation in decision-making in schools *by the pupils* whether simulated (in lessons) or for real (in school). A lot of *teacher* energy has gone into participation and decision-making—alas very often at the expense of the pupil, who may be totally excluded from this process. Indeed teachers may become so obsessed with this that their teaching may suffer. Ironically the pupils may have less real say than ever, and certainly a feeling of not being heard—yet they are the *raison d'être* of any school. What does this teach them about their futures? That the only sure way of getting attention from adults round you is to be a nuisance or to be destructive in some way? Surely the teacher's role here is to be intermediary between the pupil and the school, to interpret the one to the other. The needs of the adults too easily take over from the needs of the pupils. All this has to be worked on if schools are in any way to help their pupils become responsible mature adults.

Another difficulty schools face in relation to careers education is the number of people involved in it. Institutions like NICEC[4] are making a valiant effort to help schools co-ordinate their careers education programmes so that there are some commonly held aims and objectives for each school. It is a big step forward to find the careers teacher no longer manfully struggling on in his careers office alone. I am sure that 'careers' is a subject which should be part of the common core for all pupils, whatever their abilities and ambitions; the old idea of only giving lessons in careers to those who were leaving early is mercifully on the way out. If you involve a large number of teachers in teaching the careers programme, however, you have to spend time and energy building up a common understanding of what it is all for, and *why* it is being done. It is too easy for a desperate head teacher to timetable Miss Bloggs into the team just because she happens to have a free period when 'careers' is being taught. The whole careers programme may be invalidated if neither the teachers nor the pupils understand why they are doing it.

What about alleged pupil boredom? 'I'm not interested in becoming a nurse/engineer/deep sea diver so why bother with it?' The pupil may here be questioning a narrowly based 'square peg into square holes' approach to careers education; or conversely the teacher may be failing to convey the purpose of looking at one particular job in detail. The purpose will include consideration of the kind of personality, skills and life style which go with each job, a widening of horizons so that the pupil really does consider all factors[11] and widen his own actual range of choices. Even if he does stick to his original decision, it will be an informed decision rather than an ignorant one. Choosing a job is not really like blindman's buff, grabbing the first thing that comes along. Knowing why you *do not* want to do something is as important as realizing how much or how little real choice you actually have.

'Work experience' is another aspect of careers education which needs very careful handling. Rather like 'voluntary work' schemes, work experience can be a meaningless disaster if it is not extremely well handled. Stage one is for a school to get its pupils placed, with a great feeling of relief, for this in itself is no mean organizational feat. But what does it achieve in itself? A rush to work in that particular job because it is the only one the pupil has ever experienced at first hand? A complete rejection of that kind of work by the pupil? A hardening of the arteries of the employer *against* ever taking on pupils again? Or a genuine learning experience for pupils, employers, teachers and schools?

To achieve the latter takes an enormous amount of time. It means a dialogue between the school and the work situation. It means careful preparation of the pupils before they go out, contact and supervision when they are out, some on-going means of recording of impressions, developments and progress, some follow-up work, some feedback from the employers and from the school to the pupil and to each other. Whether the experience should be confined to one job or several, a half day a week, or a whole week at a time, or whatever: all these are vast questions which schools are usually not equipped to deal with, principally because they have still not the kind of staffing required either in quality or quantity. The argument about teachers needing to have more experience of industry is seductive but more complicated than it first seems. Teachers have been reluctant to take up the CBI 'work experience' schemes for teachers, perhaps because they know full well how destructive it is to their schools if they go away for three weeks. Many teachers, however, have worked in other settings apart from also being husbands and wives, parents, citizens, voters, ratepayers etc so their experience is not as limited as it is sometimes made to sound.

The transition from school to work is another big area which needs to be explored and worked on much more in schools.[12] The real skill in this seems to be to make opportunities for communication and interchange between schools and employers, not confrontation. The dissatisfaction of employers with the finished products of schools is already more legendary than real, as is the so-called inability of schools to deliver the goods. The problem has been that schools have been very busy delivering goods without being clear as to what they are delivering them *for*. Neither are the employers as clear about this as you would imagine from their outcries. Apart from such nonsense as employers still using imperial measures when schools went decimal years ago, I suspect that many of the difficulties arise more than anything else from the state of the economy, the stage of economic growth, and the unemployment situation. In this as in so many issues, there needs to be long, clear-headed discussion and interchange, so that at least reality and commonsense can prevail. What is hard for the teaching profession to face is the success of courses run by such agencies as the TSA in making unemployable young people employable.[13] We have to ask why this is.

The 'unemployment' situation for young people is potentially extremely depressing unless we in schools have the courage to make our pupils think about it and be prepared at least to a certain extent for this event at some stage in their lives. There are already some books around to help with this prospect.[14] It is particularly depressing that our society is so concerned with employment that to be without a job is almost like being without a name or an identity. Certainly our status as people should come from being what we are as persons and not just from our job title. Being retired, or 'only a housewife', or only a pupil/student or unemployed–these can be *positive* states, and certainly should not automatically carry the overtones of second class citizen that they so often do carry.

Another important concept in both counselling and careers education, which needs to be taken up more vigorously in schools, is the idea of education and careers development as a life-long process. The decision a pupil makes when he leaves school about what he is going to do with his future is by no means as important as we sometimes make out. Most people are going to change their jobs and the pattern of their lives several times during their lifetime. Sometimes this will be for 'reasons beyond their control', ie no more jobs in their chosen field; sometimes it will be a positive step taken by them out of deliberate choice. Whether this happens by accident or design, it can always be treated as an opportunity for growth by an adult who has a positive, confident approach to life, who is realistically aware of his strengths and weaknesses, who is able to take risks, explore new situations, cope with change and with conflict.

So what are we doing in schools to develop in our pupils these sorts of qualities? Most of our pupils, including the girls, will now have working lives of some 40 years, if they so wish. For this time-span the thought of doing one job is not only boring, it is also unrealistic. So many adults who did not enjoy school particularly blossom at a later stage in their lives and suddenly develop new interests and aptitudes, be they hobbies or jobs. So one of our tasks in school is to help our young people see themselves as whole persons, with leisure, family and community lives to lead as well as jobs to do; to help our young people realize that very few decisions about careers are irrevocable, if they are prepared to start again later; to help them know how to start again later, when they are ready; *not* to reject them out of hand if they cannot take advantage of the educational opportunities given to them when they are at school; *not* to overvalue academic achievement so that this becomes the only yardstick for 'success', for it patently is not; to use methods of teaching our young people, which enable them to grow and develop their resources, *not* methods which merely contain and control; to respect and value our pupils so that they have sufficient self-esteem to face the world; to avoid over-protecting or overpraising our pupils which may give them a false idea of their own importance and ability; to provide some experiences of stress and conflict to enable our pupils to learn to cope with these with our *support* but not our intervention; to give our pupils *genuine* opportunities for taking responsibility for their own actions and facing the consequences; *not* to iron out all the difficulties of being adolescent, but to help our pupils work at them for themselves.

To me this is what schools are about. These are counselling objectives, careers objectives, educational objectives. I hope that you will be able to see these objectives behind what I say in this book. In the next and succeeding chapters I recount in quite simple terms the work I did first as a counsellor and then as a deputy head. I have kept to the tenses I used at the time of writing. The details relate to the way things were then and what happened then. The principles upon which the work was based remain true; so do the pupils' feelings. Although what I wrote was originally geared towards the teacher who was interested in becoming a counsellor, now it seems to me that it can be usefully taken up by any adult working in a professional way with young persons on the point of growing up.

References

1. ILEA Literacy Survey 1971 (using Rutter's social adjustment scale)
2. A. Clegg and B. Megson *Children in Distress* (Penguin 1968)
3. D.H. Hamblin and A.G. Watts *Training Courses for School Counsellors* (CRAC)
4. The National Institute for Careers Education and Counselling, Bateman St, Cambridge
5. The *British Journal of Guidance and Counselling* published by CRAC (Careers Research and Advisory Centre) Cambridge
6. M. Marland *Pastoral Care* (Heinemann 1974)
7. C. Avent *Practical Approaches to Careers Education* (Hobsons Press 1974)
8. *Training Opportunities for Women* (Training Services Agency 1975)
9. (a) A. Jones, J. Marsh and A.G. Watts *Male and Female–Choosing your Role in Modern Society* (Hobsons Press 1974)
   (b) A. Jones, J. Marsh and A.G. Watts *Living Choices: Home and Family in Modern Society* (Hobsons Press 1976)
10. J. Bazalgette *School Life and Work Life in the Inner City* (in press 1977)
11. A technique promoted by Edward de Bono's thinking lessons (CORT, Cambridge)
12. M. Carter *Home, School and Work* (Pergamon 1972)
    J. Maizels *Adolescent Needs and the Transition from School to Work* (Athlone Press 1970)
13. *Vocational Preparation for Young People* (Training Services Agency 1975)
14. P. Lawrie *On the Dole* (Kogan Page 1976)

Chapter 2

The advent of the counsellor

I began my work as a school counsellor in 1965. At that time the idea of school counselling was new to Britain, so new in fact that I would often be mistaken for a kind of local politician. Friends and acquaintances who were interested in education would always begin by asking me why I was needed. What could a counsellor do that a form teacher couldn't do? Haven't British teachers always acted as counsellors and confidants to their pupils? Don't British teachers take a pride in looking after the whole pupil, not just in teaching their subject? So I shall begin with these questions.

It is true that counselling in schools is not altogether new; what is new is the establishment of the counsellor as a new professional species with professional skills. In October 1965, courses for training school counsellors (who must be trained teachers with five years' teaching experience) were set up at the Universities of Reading and Keele. Since then others have mushroomed throughout the country. The thrust from below is there, but the pull from above has yet to come. There is still no official policy, no national directive, no frame of reference, no statutory duties or powers laid down about school counselling. Counsellors have a great deal of freedom from red tape but at the same time enormous scope for damaging as well as promoting the well-being of school students.

It is therefore not surprising that the advent of the professional school counsellor should have been hailed with mixed feelings. In part this is because the counsellor's role is ill defined and badly understood. Many regard the superimposition of the counsellor on the educational structure as an unnecessary extravagance in an age when economic and academic resources are scarce. Some regard the counsellor with over-enthusiasm as a magical cure-all; some regard counselling as a bandwagon for the ambitious or unsuccessful teacher to jump on; some see the counsellor as a threat, someone making a takeover bid for the powers of the conscientious form teacher, the careers officer and the child guidance clinic. The fact that school counselling is an American import only adds to our resistance; we mark our defiance by spelling the word with a double l: counsellor, not counselor.

The subject of counselling is emotionally explosive in the educational world, triggering off conflict and ambivalence even in those who purport to sympathize with the movement. Few of us understand what the counsellor is trying to do, and even the counsellors themselves are not agreed upon this. There are probably as many different schemes of counselling in the country as there are counsellors. Indeed sceptics might be tempted to say of counselling as Eysenck has said of psychotherapy, that 'it is an unidentified technique applied to unspecified problems with unpredictable outcomes.' A natural distrust of the unknown, a fear of being made somehow to appear inadequate or diminished by the counsellor makes us all wary; it is tempting to fall back on the security of tried and tested routines, backed by economic argument, to avoid facing the immensely complicated issues and implications which the whole idea of school counsellors involves.

Any simple definition of counselling is bound to be misleading and incomplete. In chapter 3 the nature of counselling will be discussed at greater length. But it is important to any understanding of this book to attempt a definition at this stage. Basically counselling is an enabling process, designed to help an individual come to terms with his life as it is and ultimately to grow to greater maturity through learning to take responsibility and to make decisions for himself. In modern connotation, counselling is not meant to denote a process of advice-giving, of *telling* someone what to do, but rather of providing the conditions under which an individual will be able to make up his mind what, if anything, he should do. Sometimes an individual needs help of a specific nature, for example objective information about a job or about his own limitations and capabilities; sometimes he needs simply to talk out in a calm, relaxed atmosphere his innermost thoughts and conflicts. Counselling is not of course a word to be used exclusively in the school context; this is the kind of service that the Marriage Guidance Council provides through its counsellors for those with marital problems; counselling also has much in common with what social workers call casework.

In the past the role of the counsellor was fulfilled in the community spontaneously by a variety of people; the priest, the doctor, a relative, a godparent, the school master, someone who had a certain detachment or objectivity and to whom qualities of wisdom, understanding and experience were attributed. In schools these roles have always been filled intuitively by certain members of staff, not necessarily the pupil's own form teacher or house tutor, but often someone associated less with authority, perhaps a matron, an art master or a home economics mistress. The problem now is that for various reasons such as the breakdown of the extended family network and the pace and pressures of modern living, it is sometimes difficult for individuals to get help when they need it. Furthermore spontaneous intuitive counsellors, however genuine and well intentioned, may be insufficiently skilled, objective or leisured to give all the help required. At the same time that life has become more and more complex, the structure of society has become decreasingly supportive to the individual. Man's social role, moral code, the pattern of his family life, his work and his leisure are in a constant state of evolution. The Seebohm Committee's proposals[1] for the reorganization of local authority personal social services to provide a more effective community based and family orientated service recognize, by implication, the growing need of the individual to be able to get professional help with the problems, conflicts and choices which may beset him. At the same time the proposals attempt to simplify and unify the personal social services to make it easier for the individual to seek the help he may need, but so often does not know where to find.

By analogy, in schools we find mirrored the same dilemmas and complexities as in society. Teachers may be interested in helping their individual charges but they do not always have the time, the opportunity or the skills to do so fully. The reorganization of secondary schools into larger, more impersonal units makes this a good moment for rationalizing guidance services in schools. In doing this, we would be foolish indeed if we did not draw on the experience and the expertise of American school counsellors before devising a system suited to the needs of our secondary school students. For a brief overview of the situation in America, it is worth reading the NFER publication by Hugh Lytton called *School Counselling and Counsellor Education in the United States* 1968.[2]

In America the school 'counselor' has three main functions: educational guidance (help with subject choice and academic progress), vocational guidance (help in choosing or finding a job or career) and personal guidance (help with any personal problem). Counselling is really a technique used in guidance and is most relevant to personal guidance. The three threads of guidance are of course inextricably entwined, though it seems to me that this is one of the factors which makes for the semantic and practical dilemmas faced in defining the counsellor and his functions. It *is* possible to distinguish between vocational guidance (which is closely linked with educational guidance) and personal guidance, or counselling. A person who comes for vocational guidance may need counselling at a personal level before he can make an objective decision, but not necessarily so. It is asking a lot of a counsellor to expect him to combine the great technical knowledge of job content and opportunities, skill in testing, slotting, evaluating and recording abilities required of the educational/vocational counsellor, with the much more passive yet exacting role of personal counsellor. What may happen when the two roles are combined is that the counsellor is not able, through lack of time, to fulfil his non-evaluative, non-directive listening role. The more direct vocational guidance role, with its tangible results in the shape of record cards and decisions, may take over. Anyone who attempts vocational guidance should be acquainted with and be able to use counselling techniques; indeed vocational counsellors *should* use counselling techniques, but because of pressures of time they may not always be able to counsel as much as they would wish or as much as their clients need. All school students need vocational guidance; only a small proportion need personal counselling, but for this small proportion it is very important for their future well-being that their needs are not overlooked.

The relevance of this to the situation in Britain is clear. Behind the movement for the introduction of counselling into British schools are the two complementary but different threads with their different motives. On the one hand there is the entirely justifiable desire of those concerned with occupational guidance for the young to provide a better service. The counsellor would appear a ready-made vehicle for such a service, thus helping to avoid any more wastage of educational ability (see Robbins and Crowther Reports[3,4]) and helping young people find more interesting and skilled jobs which, it is presumed, would bring them greater self-fulfilment and happiness. On the other hand there is the mental health movement which, under the auspices of the National Association for Mental Health, set up in 1963 a working party to look into the needs of young people for counselling.[5] This movement sees counselling as a supplement to the school mental health/social welfare services, rather than as a booster to the economic health of the nation, though of course the two aspects are linked. Under the umbrella of the mental health movement come schemes for education in personal relationships, some of which are run by the Marriage Guidance Council, some of which teachers themselves undertake, possibly after training by the Marriage Guidance Council.

Existing university courses for counsellors are broad based, seeming to fit their counsellors for any eventuality.[6] Any analysis of what existing counsellors actually do shows that they encompass a wide range of functions. What may be happening is that, in order to sell his services, the counsellor has to compromise himself by doing a little of everything, including teaching, or being senior master. By doing a little of everything he may well do himself out of existence, and simply be in effect a teacher like any other, who happens to have an advanced diploma in education and might therefore be expected to take extra responsibility. But if we are to have school counsellors as such in Britain, it must not be simply because they exist, but because they are necessary, that is to say, because they are fulfilling some essential function in school which is not and cannot be provided by any other service.

Guidance services in British schools

Let us look now at this problem the other way round, and examine the provision in English schools for educational, vocational and personal guidance. It is true that there does already exist in our schools a team of people who compositely fulfil, at least in theory, the functions of the American counsellor and more. Most of the responsibility for guidance lies in fact with the form teacher. He in turn is supported and directed in his work by the house or year master and the headmaster. When necessary he can call on the services of the educational psychologist, the careers officer and the education welfare officer to provide the supplementary specialist skills and knowledge he lacks.

The English system of diffused responsibility for guidance has the merits of providing an elaborate network of care for the individual and of making use of whatever talents in this respect that the staff may have. The snag is that it is an amateur system and a random system. It depends on the inspired intuitive gifts of the teacher, and is based on the assumption that all teachers are gifted in this direction, which is patently not always the case. True, it provides safeguards for the individual: the house master can make up for deficiencies in the form tutor, and the head can provide support for the house master. But it is the form tutor who is fundamentally in the key position here and this important fact is not always realized or accepted. Reorganization of schools into larger comprehensive units means that heads have to delegate more to house masters who in turn must delegate to form tutors. But effective delegation has to include some specification of the role and duties involved in 'pastoral care' and some training for this role. How often is this thoroughly done?

If we were to do a job analysis of the form teacher's functions, we would find that the form teacher makes of his job what he will, according to his age, aptitude and ability. Dinner money is taken, registers are marked, attendance slips are filled in, reports are produced on time, but over and above these tangible tasks is a whole range of activity which may or may not take place.

Pastoral care is a vague concept. While most form teachers provide a high standard of pastoral care, it is also true that some teachers have little interest in this aspect of their work, and some have little talent for it, even though they may be interested in it: notwithstanding these may all be good teachers. All form tutors, whatever their intuitive skills, could be helped to be more effective, more perceptive and more objective in their approach to their charges if their initial training prepared them more thoroughly for this role, and if they regularly discussed their role and their problems in groups within schools. Schemes of this kind do exist, but not as a part of standard educational practice. Those interested in the training of teachers through groups should read Elizabeth Richardson's sensitive account of her work in the Department of Education at Bristol, *Group Study for Teachers.*[7]

Training in professional skills, for heads, house masters and teachers alike, should include experience in groups to bring a heightened awareness of the emotional forces at play in any school situation. It should also include study and experience of interview techniques, with particular emphasis on the art of listening, and an understanding of counselling techniques.

Educational guidance

In many British secondary schools educational guidance is undertaken by house masters in conjunction with form tutors. By educational guidance I mean not only help with choice of subjects but also the maintenance of systematic and objective records of a student's attainment and development.

Pupils arrive at secondary school with a primary school profile which may form the beginning of their secondary school record card, and which usually gives an objective measurement or grade for certain abilities. We do not normally ask the secondary teacher to give individual tests of intelligence and attainment; this is the job of the educational psychologist, who will test children at the request of the school in cases where the teacher suspects either that a pupil's work is falling below its potential or that a pupil is strained because he is pushing himself beyond his capabilities. Whether the educational psychologist is used in this testing capacity as much as he might be depends on a number of factors: whether the psychologist himself believes in tests, how busy the psychologist is with 'more serious' cases, how aware the teacher is of the existence of such a service, how much confidence the teacher has in putting forward a problem case. Many teachers find real difficulty in deciding when a child needs educational testing and therefore only ask for it in extreme cases when they are absolutely sure of themselves, and not afraid either of making themselves look ridiculous or of wasting the psychologist's time. A lot of us feel rather the same about doctors: it is not enough that they provide a service, we must be confident enough to use it.

This line of argument assumes that objective measurement of ability is an important component in educational guidance. Not everyone would agree that it is. There are certainly moments in a pupil's school career when such impartial information would be invaluable. For example, if pupils have to choose between courses, it is relevant to know whether this pupil is potentially university, college of education, A level, O level or CSE material, or whether he had best follow a vocational or general course. But an experienced teacher will claim here that he is able to tell where a pupil's abilities place him in the spectrum of choice, and he may well be right. He will also claim that the pupil may not have reached his full potential yet, and that to make a rigid cut-off point would be unfair. Certainly a form teacher who has known both pupil and staff over a period of time will understand more than any outsider the true meaning of a B+ for Miss Smith in geography and a C+ for Mr Burns in mathematics. But it is possible to make a mistake in placing even though a school's policy may be to keep course choice as revocable and flexible as possible. The important point here, surely, is to spot the under achievers, to find out why they are under achievers and to help them to fulfil their potential.

Devising more sophisticated record cards and keeping them properly filled in are tasks which could be allotted to a school counsellor and take up a lot of his time. But before we embark upon such a scheme we have to ask why we need record cards; if we need them, how can we best ensure that they are to be useful, and if they are to be useful, who should keep them. There is no reason why heads, advised by educational psychologists, should not devise effective records schemes to be filled in by form teachers; indeed this is what already often happens. In other words, more sophisticated educational guidance mechanisms are important topics to be considered in the running of comprehensive schools, but they are not conclusive arguments for the introduction of school counsellors.

Whoever is responsible for guiding the pupil with his choices, be he house master, form tutor or counsellor, needs to remember that a student likes to feel he has had some say in the matter, and is more likely to work hard at a subject he has chosen than at a subject he has had thrust upon him.

Vocational guidance

Decisions made through educational guidance do of course have vital implications for vocational guidance and this is why it is so important for these inseparable processes to be continuous and on-going throughout a child's school life. Crisis-counselling of school leavers is generally regarded by the careers service as an unsatisfactory process of limited value. Thorough vocational guidance involves not just careers advisers, whoever they may be, but the whole education of the individual. More attention needs to be given not just to providing more information about jobs at an earlier stage but also to providing more opportunity for schoolchildren to make decisions and, most subtle of all, to motivating them to want to study, stay on, do well. And we must remember that it is not enough to motivate the children if their parents do not share these aspirations. These I think are points which teachers are in a position to influence more than counsellors. Whatever the answers to these problems—and there is no simple solution—it is certain that there is need and scope for better vocational guidance in schools. If we accept this we then have to decide whether it should be provided by the all-purpose counsellor, by a specialist occupational counsellor, by a school based careers officer, or by a careers teacher. But the person who takes on this role will have to spend a lot of time working with form tutors and house masters to ensure that they understand, share and help to implement what he is trying to do.

Personal guidance

What about the provision of personal guidance under our existing system of pastoral care? Like the other types of guidance, its provision is patchy, not sufficiently structured into the official fabric of school life and dependent in quality very largely on the attitudes and personality of the head, house staff and form tutors. The official organs of personal guidance for students at risk are the child guidance clinics for psychological problems and the welfare services, notably the social services, for social problems. In many areas these services are not able to do as much preventive work as they would like for a number of reasons. These are community services and parents who are worried can make direct and confidential contact with them, but parents do not always know this. Heads too are sometimes insufficiently informed about the nature and purpose of the services and sceptical of their value: the research in the Plowden Report on this topic, although done in primary schools, is probably relevant here.[8] Both services, particularly the school psychological services, are understaffed (see the Seebohm Report and the Summerfield Report[9]). Most child guidance clinics either have a waiting list, or schools think they have a waiting list and therefore hesitate to use them. In any case problem children are often referred when their problems have reached such magnitude that the pupils concerned are disrupting in some way the smooth functioning of school life. Teachers may find it difficult to decide when a child's behaviour requires the attention of a psychiatrist and hesitate to approach the educational psychologist for a second opinion in the same way that they may hesitate to approach him about testing: that is unless they are very confident, unless the head is particularly sympathetic to the psychological services and unless the psychologist is known to the staff, liked by the staff and seen to perform a useful function either by referring children to the child guidance clinic or by counselling children and their parents. At a time when educational psychologists are in such short supply, they are simply not in school often enough to advise and reassure a member of staff with an embryonic problem child. This is where the counsellor could be useful.

Theoretically the education welfare officer is the person who can advise the head about social welfare services and which agency to use. The Plowden Report research here again shows the education welfare officer service to be understaffed both in quality and quantity and that its former role of 'attendance officer' looms large. Heads may be lucky enough to have an outstanding welfare officer attached to their schools; if not they have to depend on their own knowledge of the social services and their own contacts with them, which may be very good or may be minimal. What is more, whatever information heads manage to glean about the present tangle of social welfare services is not always passed on to the form teacher. Teachers may not often have the opportunity for contact with outside welfare agencies and their knowledge of them may become theoretical and clouded. Obvious social problems are dealt with, but is this enough? Could more preventive work be done in schools?

The form tutor

Let us look for a moment at an 'ideal' form tutor: sensitive, aware of his own limitations, he has the interests of his pupils uppermost in his mind, without getting over-involved in their problems; he is constantly aware of the emotional undercurrents in his form and able to forestall problems before they develop; he does not hesitate to ask advice from his house master or head, and he brings in experts such as educational psychologists and careers officers at the earliest opportunity. He thus combines the best in guidance with a balanced overall view of the pupil and continuity of care.

Many form tutors achieve all this and more; many understandably fall short of this ideal. Most heads learn quickly to accept the limitations of their staff, to make the best of the qualities their staff do have by a subtle balance of staff characteristics throughout each academic year and an intricate network of safeguards, provided through other personnel such as house masters, to see that individual pupils suffer as little as possible. But what happens when heads have practically no choice of form tutor? With the present numbers of part-time teachers in schools, it is likely that heads will have to use most remaining full-time staff as form tutors, yet not all of these will be entirely enthusiastic about or suited for this role.

Continuity of care is another myth which befuddles our thinking about the role of the form teacher. Some schools as a matter of policy institute continuity of care in an attempt to counterbalance effects of size and impersonality. Thus a child may keep the same house master all his school life and the same form teacher for two or three years at a time. The system breaks down when staff turnover is high, and when there is a basic clash of personality between the individual pupil and the person in charge of him throughout his school life. There is no simple way out of this dilemma: the important principle is to structure the system of pastoral care so that an individual child has a choice of adults with whom to relate who know him sufficiently well to see him in perspective. Thus a blockage in a relationship with one teacher or the sudden departure of another would not leave a child either feeling victimized or thinking that nobody really knows him or cares for him.

If we accept that form teachers could improve the quality of the pastoral care they provide if they were given more specific training for this role, and if they had both knowledge and experience of counselling techniques, we must also accept that it is unlikely even then that they would be able to serve all the needs of every individual in their care. We have to face even in the most outstanding form teacher limitations placed upon him by his other roles. His first job after all is to teach and he does not have time to be all things to all his form members. Furthermore his other roles in the structure of the school community may limit his counselling potential in the eyes of his pupils.

First the question of time. Form tutors are normally given very little free time with their form. Some may not even teach all the members of their form and their contact with them may be therefore limited to morning and afternoon registration. Occasionally schools establish 'form periods' to help overcome this particular problem, but often this kind of form time is spent in a rather embarrassed way in quizzes, debates and just doing homework. Few form teachers systematically interview every member of their form at regular intervals and contact with parents is even more haphazard. A child will be summoned for interview by form or house tutor normally only in certain prescribed circumstances: if the child is in trouble, if he is to be sent on an errand or asked to perform some duty, if he is to be asked for some information.

Let us suppose that the child wishes to talk about something that is bothering him. First he has to pluck up the courage to make an approach, and this in itself is not easy. Unless a specific time is set aside for the interview, it is quite possible that the child will not be able to get round to his real problem because the bell for the next lesson has gone and teacher and child alike have a duty to move on. Moreover it takes an exceptionally perceptive or unharassed teacher to see that a simple statement may be the cue for a need for a longer chat.

Take for example the statement: 'My sister's having a baby tomorrow.' A busy teacher might reply, 'How nice for you. Would you mind sitting down while I take the register?' A less harassed teacher will ask a few questions about it and remember to ask a few more after the baby is born. But what the child may really need is not for someone to ask her questions, but someone to *listen* to her. What she may really need is to express her own fears and worries about childbirth, her own insecurity and ambivalence in the face of this new rival within the family. To be able to do this the pupil needs to talk to someone who is not in a hurry, who is giving all his attention to the interview and who is not worrying about the fact that he is late for his next lesson and that there will be a rumpus in the classroom. There is no reason why the form teacher should not suggest a meeting during lunch hour or after school to continue the discussion, but unless this is a recognized, expected and established pattern of school procedure, it is unlikely to be either suggested or used to any great extent. In any case, teachers often have staff meetings of various kinds after school and little 'free' time.

There are other factors too which may block the possibility of real communication between form teacher and form pupil. The form teacher's duty to look after his form is subordinate in fact to his duty to teach his subject and his duty to see that the children in his charge keep the school rules and regulations, work hard and do not waste time. The strength of the teacher's authoritarian role will depend on how democratically the school is run, and how tolerant and permissive is the teacher's basic personality. But however flexible and fearless the teacher, he will still have to demand conformity from his pupils on certain points, whatever his beliefs, if he is to do his job. He is likely in any case to be perceived by his pupils as an instrument of authority; indeed if he is not perceived in this way he may be doing a disservice to schools, pupils and himself alike by undermining the school disciplinary system. But because of the teacher's authority, his role as a potential counsellor may have certain limits. Rebels and drop-outs may find it particularly hard to turn to him either because he stands for what they oppose or because they realize his more liberal tendencies but do not want to put him in a dilemma. Children recognize, sometimes more than we credit, the limitations of our roles.

Another factor which may block the form teacher's counselling potential is his judgemental role. Teachers are constantly asked to make judgements on their pupils by assessing their academic work, their industriousness, their behaviour, their potential and their personality. True there is in many schools a swing away from percentages and positions but it is important for the school, the pupil and his parents to have some idea of the progress the pupil is making, both in relation to his own potential and by comparison with his peers. Assessments of behaviour or personality are bound to reflect the teacher's own attitudes and prejudices. Pupils are therefore not going to reveal to teachers, unless they can help it, information that may be damaging to their image and prejudicial to their reputations.

The same sort of behaviour is to be observed in the relationship between any employee and his boss; in the school situation between the teacher and the head, and between parent and head too. 'Such a good teacher,' the head may say, in all sincerity. 'She takes such an interest in her children.' Or 'Such a good mother; she understands her daughter so well.' This may not be how the child concerned feels.

Most of us present some kind of façade to those in authority over us. We may do this consciously or unconsciously. When we break through the façade, it is either because we trust the person concerned enough to know they will not hold it against us, or because we have ceased to care what they think about us. Clearly parents and form teachers should know their children well enough to see through the outer image, simply because they have contact with them every day. But this conclusion does not necessarily follow; unless we are emotionally disturbed and our feelings are so strong that we can no longer control them, most of us reserve the horrors of our innermost thoughts for those few people we can trust sufficiently not to use them in evidence against us or our families.

So although children may need to talk to someone, they may not turn to their teacher, not only because they perceive the teacher's judgemental role. Another factor may be that they cannot be sure that what they tell in confidence will be kept confidential. Children recognize that teachers are liable to react to pieces of confidential information like most other human beings. Either they will want to pass this information on, because they feel it important to know everything about the child; or they will want to act upon this information because it provokes in them anxieties of their own and feelings of concern for the child which can only be dissipated by 'doing something'. For example a child might tell a teacher that her parents are unhappily married, that her mother once had an affair with a Negro and that her father beats her mother up every Friday. Supposing this information to be true, all it tells you about *the child* is that she is worried and that she needs, at this moment, a little extra sympathy and support, and a chance to talk over her feelings. Once she has done this the relevance of the information to an understanding of the child is diminished; if such information became common knowledge among the staff it could lead to a stereotyping of the image of the child's family and a distortion of the child's own image which would do nothing to help her. Or supposing a child confides that her father has been making incestuous advances towards her. If this is true and incest has taken place, then it is a case for the law. If it is not true, but really a fantasy in the child's mind, built upon her own desires, then premature action can only make matters worse. Clearly a child in this situation needs a lot of help, but the help must come from someone with professional skills for dealing with such a situation.

COMMENT. We can gain immensely from a study of American counselling theory and practice, but any British system of school counselling must be based on the needs of our particular social and educational structure. Counsellors must either provide a service which does not exist and which is regarded as essential or they must replace or combine the functions of other personnel as part of the trend, reflected in the community, of simplifying and unifying personal social services as society becomes organized in larger units. If we look at existing school guidance services we see that *educational guidance* is at present undertaken by house masters and form tutors who could be helped by more training to improve their skills for this role. There is relatively little choice of subject within most schools' curricula. Educational psychologists can be used for educational testing, or more teachers trained to do this work. *Vocational guidance* is not sufficiently linked with educational guidance and motivation. The careers service has not at the moment adequate supplies of skilled manpower to provide an occupational counsellor for each large school. We have to decide whether to train counsellors for this specific role or simply increase the size of the careers service. In the area of *personal guidance* not all teachers have talents for helping individuals with their problems and those who do could improve their techniques of pastoral care with more training and self-awareness. Form teachers have considerable potential as counsellors but there are limits to their counselling role partly because of their other roles in the structure of the school and partly because they have so little spare time. Normal children do nevertheless have a need at times to form a relationship and to talk out their problems and conflicts with an adult who can listen sympathetically and respect their confidences and whose role is in no way either authoritarian or judgemental.

References

1. *Report of the Committee on Local Authority and Allied Personal Social Services* the Seebohm Report (HMSO 1968)
2. H. Lytton *School Counselling and Counsellor Education in the US* (NFER 1968)
3. *Higher Education* the Robbins Report (HMSO 1963)
4. *15 to 18* the Crowther Report (HMSO 1959)
5. *Working Party Report on Counselling Services in Schools* (National Association for Mental Health 1969)
6. *Counselling in Schools* Schools Council working paper no 15 (HMSO 1967)
7. E. Richardson *Group Study for Teachers* (Routledge and Kegan Paul 1967)
8. *Children and Their Primary Schools* the Plowden Report (HMSO 1967)
9. *Psychologists in Education Services* the Summerfield Report (HMSO 1968)

Chapter 3

What is counselling?

In this chapter I want to discuss the meaning and nature of counselling at greater length. Although many teachers now recognize that some individual students need more help than they can provide in the time available to them, others postulate gloomily a kind of Parkinson's law of counselling: adolescent problems expand to occupy the number of counsellors available. Leave adolescents alone, they say, and their problems will sort themselves out with the fullness of time. Is this so? Is counselling simply a soft option for the malingering drop-out? The truth is that counselling is not all that comfortable a process, since it demands searching self-examination. Any counsellor worth his salt should be able to recognize when he is being abused, rather than used. Furthermore he will expect his clients to come as much from the good and the brave as from the bad and the ugly: the adolescents who are most at risk are not always the ones who show it most.

Many teachers remain confused about the nature of counselling. This is hardly surprising when so many different kinds of people claim to be counsellors. Counselling is fashionable, and that for a start puts some people off it. Teachers, doctors, social workers, psychologists, youth leaders, marriage guiders and ministers of religion all lay claim to the counselling role. Whether in fact they really do counsel, or merely think they do, will depend on many factors. The kind of help called counselling may in fact range from advice-giving to psychotherapy. The school counsellor may sometimes give advice, though this is no justification for his existence since teachers give advice very readily. Equally he may occasionally work at a psychotherapeutic level, though he would be unwise to attempt this without himself being expertly guided. But his basic role is somewhere between these two extremes. Leona Tyler has defined the aim of psychotherapy as personality change.[1] The school counsellor is more concerned with the development of what is, than with fundamental change; with the here and now more than with the deep and distant past; with making the best of a situation as it actually is, rather than with altering the way of the world. If anything changes through counselling, it is not the fabric of the client's life and personality so much as his feelings and his attitudes towards himself and others, and his degree of acceptance of himself and the world he lives in.

Adolescents in school and in society have to face many problems of adjustment and identity;[2] they have to learn to be independent, to make decisions for themselves, to take responsibility, to weather a crisis, sometimes to live with a difficult situation. Most adolescents survive this stormy period much strengthened by their experience and without needing to talk to a counsellor about their problems. The counsellor's role is to give support to those adolescents who *do* feel insecure, threatened, overwhelmed, misunderstood, unsure of their role, undecided about what they should do, and who *do* ask for help. The counsellor's role is not to cover over the adolescent's difficulties, but to help him face his problems and grow to greater maturity through them. Thus the foundation of a more integrated and balanced adulthood may be laid. School counselling is therefore appropriate for adolescents who are basically sound in mind and body, but who need help at certain stages of their development. This is not to say that their problems are not serious or real. Conflict may cause depression or despair in an adolescent, which may prevent him from taking action or being decisive, or doing his school work properly. But the problem is only part of a passing phase in the adolescent's growth and situation; it is a transitory developmental or situational problem, not a fundamental impairment of his personality.

A simple illustration might make this point clearer. June may be feeling bewildered and hurt because her mother has married again. June cannot accept her stepfather in her deceased father's role. As a result she is moping about at home and being defiant at school. She is not developing interests and activities with friends of her own age, she is doing nothing to help herself out of this despondency and she is rejecting her mother's efforts to help her. It is no good telling June to pull herself together. She will not be able to pull herself together until she has come to terms with her feelings, understood what has happened, realized that no fairy godmother is going to alter the situation and accepted that no one is trying to hurt *her*—her parents desperately want her to be happy; and that it is in her power to make the best or the worst of this situation. A sense of perspective will not come until June feels secure in herself and in the people she needs; this security may not come until she has expressed her violent feelings. She may be afraid to express her anger to her mother in case she loses her altogether. The counsellor's role is to provide the conditions in which June can begin to express her real self. The counsellor does not tell her to be sensible, to take a grip on herself. The counsellor is not trying to repair an inability to make relationships with people, because up to this time June has not found this difficult. The counsellor is simply trying to help June release and use her own resources for coping with life and take some constructive action on her own behalf. But June does *have* resources of her own; she is *capable* of taking action. Through taking responsibility herself, June develops and strengthens her ability to cope with difficult situations, an ability which will stand her in good stead when she is an adult. She has not buried her problem only to have it re-occur at a later stage in a different form, perhaps when she marries or has her first child. She has not had her problem solved by someone else, which would prevent her learning how to solve problems. Through her relationship with her counsellor she has faced her problem, she has worked through her feelings and she has learnt something useful about herself and the world.

Theories of counselling

There is a vast body of American literature on counselling theory and technique, which is best read at first hand. *Theories of Counseling* and *Techniques of Counseling* summarize the basic schools of thought in these fields, and give useful references.[3,4]

The main debate between the American theorists concerns the amount of direction the counsellor should give the content of the interview. It is generally agreed that the quality of the relationship between counsellor and client is of fundamental importance; that among the goals of counselling are 'self-understanding, self-awareness, self-acceptance, self-determination'. But are these goals best achieved by non-directive, directive or eclectic counselling techniques? *Non-directive counsellors,* inspired by the work of Carl Rogers,[5,6] put the onus of direction very much on the individual; the client must be allowed to talk about what he wants to talk about. The relationship between the counsellor and his client is in itself therapeutic and brings the freedom for the client to make his own decisions and grow towards maturity. *Directive counsellors* are more purposeful. They lead the client through an examination of his problem, go through the possible consequences of various courses of action, help the client try out various new solutions. The client is still making the decisions but the choice is largely directed by the experience and the expertise of the counsellor.[7] *Eclectic counsellors* use whatever method they feel best suits the needs of the client, arguing that some pupils, because of their age, inexperience or personality, need more specific help in making a decision than others.[8] These three types of counselling are discussed in some detail in *Client-centered Counseling in the Secondary School.*[9] More recently client problems have been seen as learning problems and the counsellor's job has been defined as 'helping his client learn more effective ways of solving his own problems'; that is, to learn more adaptive and constructive modes of behaviour.[10]

I know from my own experience how confusing it can be for a

teacher, first to come across the highly technical literature about counselling theory, second to try to reconcile these philosophies with his own philosophy and personality, third to integrate what he has learnt in theory with what he does and is in practice. We must not forget that, in fact, theories of counselling have much in common and their differences are mostly in emphasis. They have as their basis the interaction between two people, one of whom is trying to help the other. With what purpose, by which means and with what effect will depend above all on the personalities of the two persons concerned and to a lesser extent on theories and techniques. Ultimately the counsellor functions not according to a book, but according to himself, yet in a disciplined, informed and professional manner.

The elements in a counselling relationship

Let us turn now to a consideration of some of the ingredients which make up the relationship between the counsellor and his client. These ingredients are not exclusive to a counselling relationship: they might be found in any relationship between two individuals, and the fact that they are often missing is at the root of many problems between people. In family life, at work and in school, we are more likely to thrive if our relationships with the people near to us are based on mutual liking, trust, respect, tolerance and genuine concern. In the school setting the kind of relationship which exists between head and pupils, teachers and pupils, teachers and teachers, pupils and pupils, teachers and parents, affects not only the atmosphere of the school, but the amount of education that goes on. It is a sobering thought to recall how often, not intentionally, but because we are not thinking about what we are doing, we unwittingly crush instead of encourage, criticize instead of praise, belittle instead of believe, advise instead of listen, co-exist instead of communicate. Although we may not all be counsellors, or want to be counsellors, we can all learn from a consideration of what is involved in a counselling relationship.

Rapport

First there must *be* a relationship between the counsellor and his client. That might sound self-evident, but it is possible for two people to be together, to be talking, without there being any communication of feeling between them. The plays of Pinter and N.F. Simpson for example illustrate vividly some extreme cases of non-interaction. It takes time for a relationship to be established between counsellor and client, but they may quickly make rapport with each other, that is, recognize that there is, in their response to each other, a basis for building up a relationship. But for a fruitful relationship to be established, the client must want a relationship with the counsellor, and the counsellor must want to help the client, and feel that he can help him. Let us suppose for example that John is sent for counselling (by his house master) because he is unruly, aggressive and rude. If John himself either does not want or does not see the need for any help from anybody, then the counsellor may not be able to form a helpful relationship with John. He may after a while, if he is sufficiently skilled or lucky, inspire enough confidence in John for him to change his mind. But counselling will not really begin until John admits his need. If John has decided that he needs help, but the counsellor appears bored or disinterested in what he is saying, if the counsellor is thinking, 'What a dreadful type. I can quite see why no one can handle him. How on earth can I be expected to do anything with a case like this?' then there is not a sound basis for a counselling relationship. John will sense the lack of confidence and respect in the counsellor, and will not feel the warmth, trust and security in the relationship which he needs to be able to talk about how he really feels: to be able to admit for example that behind his aggressive defiance he feels unsure of himself, unloved and unwanted.

Respect for the individual

It is important that the counsellor should recognize John as an individual, as a person in his own right, and not by a stereotyped tag such as 'that long-haired lout in 5.E' or 'Brian's naughty brother' or 'one of that gang that wrecks everyone's lessons'. Recognition as an individual implies a uniqueness which is important to a sense of individual worth and self-respect. The counsellor can communicate this by showing respect for John: by being punctual and courteous, by calling John by name and by remembering the details of what John has already told him. It is insulting to John if the counsellor has to rummage through masses of notes in order to recall him, or if the counsellor confuses him with somebody else or asks about something John has already explained. The counsellor must stop and make time to review details of John's case before the interview if he cannot trust his memory; though if the counsellor does forget, it is better for him to explain than to pretend. The relationship must be as genuine as possible.

Acceptance

It is vital for the counsellor to accept the client as he is, warts and all, not only on certain conditions. If we look at John again, we see that part of his problem is that his mother is always saying, in effect, 'I won't love you unless you do as I say.' The teachers have been saying the same thing in their way, withdrawing rewards unless certain conditions are met. 'You won't go on this outing unless you behave' or 'I can't have you in this class unless you keep quiet.' This is reasonable enough for the sake of the class as a whole, but it is not going to cure John's behaviour, and is more likely to have the effect of reinforcing his sense of failure and worthlessness. The aim of the counsellor is to hold nothing against John, in no way to judge or prejudge him. He takes John as he is, without either condoning or criticizing his various misdemeanours. But the acceptance must be genuine, and come from within the counsellor. John will not be deceived if the counsellor is inwardly shocked, sceptical or suspicious. But if John feels genuine acceptance from the counsellor, he will feel less threatened by the interview situation; he will become less defensive and some of the blocks to the communication of feeling will be removed.

Empathy

The kind of response which John needs from the counsellor is called empathy, which must be distinguished from sympathy and pity. Feeling sorry for John can have the effect of making him feel more sorry for himself, which is not constructive. Sympathy is a self-centred emotion: the counsellor knows how he would feel if his mother didn't love him, but how does that help John? John needs empathy: the counsellor tries to understand how John feels in this situation. He understands John's feelings of hostility, despair, aggression, anxiety, defiance and guilt and John feels that he understands or that he really is trying to understand.

Trust

John is not going to tell the counsellor much unless he trusts him. A counsellor who is not trustworthy will have a bad reputation among the pupils, and this will undermine all that he is trying to do. Even if the counsellor is generally liked, trusted and respected by the pupils, John has to be sure for himself that the counsellor is trustworthy. This means that at first he will not tell the counsellor very much, and if the counsellor presses for intimate truths, he may meet with rebuff. First the relationship between John and his counsellor has to be established, the counsellor tested out. The counsellor has to reassure John as to who he is, why he is there, what the expectations and the limits of their relationship are. He has to do this in a way which John can understand, that is without recourse to psychological terminology, which could either be incomprehensible or intimidating. John must know for example that if he says his mother is lazy and selfish, the counsellor will not pass this on to his mother: to do this would damage John's relationship with his mother, and the aim of the counselling is quite the opposite–to improve this relationship.

Both the counsellor and John realize that these statements are only partially true, that they express John's despair and anger at his mother's inability to reassure him of her love. Similarly John must know that the counsellor will not pass on this information to the teaching staff because, in fact, John loves his mother very much and does not want to blacken her name; he needs to express his hostility towards her to someone he can trust, but that is all. John also needs to be able to say that he hates school, that he cannot tolerate this teacher, that it is all unfair; but he must trust the counsellor not to pass this on to the school; otherwise his life there will become even more intolerable. John has to trust the counsellor sufficiently to start to ventilate his true feelings before he can begin to get his problem into perspective: when he has done this, he may be ready to consider his own part in it all and to what extent his own attitudes, his own expectations of others and of himself and his own behaviour are influencing his life.

Confidentiality

One of the first points the counsellor must explain to John then is the principle of confidentiality. He must make it clear that he will not pass on to anyone anything which is told him in confidence without John's agreement. This must include not only sensational facts like the time John found his mother in bed with his 'uncle' Bob, but feelings, like John's deprecatory attitudes to those in authority over him. (The staff know about those already, but there is no need for the counsellor to reinforce their hostility towards John.) However John will not be helped unless something of what he is feeling is communicated to his parents and his teachers. Ideally John will undertake this himself and then there are no problems of misrepresentation. But often John will need the help of the counsellor in doing this; the counsellor can pave the way for a more sympathetic reception of the new improved John. So the counsellor may say to John, 'I think it might be helpful for your teacher to know that you are finding life at home rather a strain, particularly as your father is away.' If John agrees but does not want to talk about it himself, the counsellor gets his permission to talk this over with the form teacher. The permission to talk is part of the respect shown by the counsellor for John. The form teacher says that he knew already that John had problems at home: yes, it must be very hard for a strong virile young man like John not to see his father; mother seemed to be finding it very hard to cope the last time John was in trouble and she was sent for by the head. Perhaps we need to handle John in a different way? The counsellor does not tell the teacher what to do, but tries to harness his sympathy for and understanding of John, feelings which have rather disappeared in the strain and exasperation of dealing with him daily.

What about seeing mother? Again there is no doubt that this can be extremely valuable to the counsellor, both to gain greater insight into John and to assess his problems realistically and also to help the mother to think more of John's point of view. But is it valuable to John? Only if John agrees that this would be helpful. If the interview is against his will, then it will destroy the bond of trust and respect between him and the counsellor; it will cause alienation not communication. If John agrees to the interview, the counsellor may find that both before and after John needs reassuring that the interview was in his best interests, and not a part of a new alliance of mother and counsellor against him.

Supposing during the course of counselling John tells the counsellor that he has 'got a girl into trouble' and that she is under the age of consent. Where a law has been broken, or where there is moral or physical danger to an individual, then the counsellor has a duty to society, the school and John's family to consider. It is only fair for the counsellor to make this clear at the very outset, so that if John tells him about this, he knows that action may be taken: perhaps this is what John wants and all he is asking for is some courage in facing up to his responsibilities in this. With the counsellor's support John may be able himself to tell the appropriate persons what has happened and face the consequences of his action or he may ask the counsellor to help him communicate the truth. But this can be done discreetly and tactfully by involving only those people who really need to know about this incident, avoiding publicity and panic and thus retaining John's dignity as far as possible. He is punishable within the law, but there is no need to make a public scapegoat of him as well. Indeed if John gains the strength to shoulder his responsibility the incident can be turned to constructive rather than destructive use. But before the counsellor does anything at all about this particular kind of incident, not only does he get John's agreement but he makes perfectly sure that this *is* the truth and not something John has made up because of his great need to demonstrate his manliness. If it is true but John refuses to give permission for action to be taken, then the counsellor may feel he has a duty to society to act nevertheless; but again as a mark of his respect for John he does not do this without first telling John what he is going to do and why. In my experience it has never been necessary to go against a child's wishes in this sort of case. Each case has to be judged on its merits and the point at which the counsellor feels conflict between his duty to society and his duty to the boy will depend on the disposition of the counsellor and the terms of reference under which he is working. The unattached youth worker may feel more freedom than the counsellor working within an institution. There is no golden rule, but it is my belief that the counsellor should make clear his legal and ethical position at the outset, so that someone like John is not lulled into revealing all and then is 'shopped'. This is unethical and untenable. The counsellor is not a spy service for the authorities and his first duty is to the individual child. The counsellor has therefore to be sufficiently strong in himself not to have to relieve his own anxiety or pass the buck of responsibility by taking premature unnecessary or unethical action. But it should be very rare indeed for the counsellor not to get the co-operation of his client.

Testing

Suppose during counselling it emerges that John would like to know whether he is capable of going to university, and a psychological test may be useful. John has asked for this because he has already grown to the point where he can take constructive action on his own behalf. Some counsellors prefer not to undertake testing themselves, even under these conditions; they feel that psychological testing is likely to hinder the progress of the counselling relationship, by putting the counsellor in an evaluating judgemental role, which may inhibit the client's freedom to express his feelings; they regard testing as the job of the educational psychologist or psychometrist. Whoever administers the test, its purpose is to help the client; the information obtained by the counsellor is for the use of the client himself. There is obviously a place for testing in schools, but not necessarily within the counselling relationship unless the client wants it.

The counselling interview

What is the counsellor doing during his interviews with John? Basically he is listening. This is not as easy as it sounds. The teacher exhausted from chalk and talk might think enviously of the counsellor sitting listening in a cosy one-to-one relationship. It is easier in one way only: the counsellor is giving his attention to the needs of one person instead of 20 or 30, and he is not trying to teach facts as well as encourage the weak, stimulate the strong and discipline the unruly. But the quality of the listening relationship between the counsellor and his client is at a deeper and therefore more demanding level than any classroom interaction; and there is no respite, none of the mechanical tasks such as setting homework or giving out books, none of the changes of tempo such as posing a problem for the class to solve in groups, which bring in the classroom the necessary breathing space for the teacher to gather together his thoughts and his strength.

When the counsellor is listening to John, he needs to give his full attention, body and soul, all the time. He is not just listening to what John is saying, he is trying to feel the feelings behind the words and he is observing the way John is sitting and looking. Nails being bitten, fingers tapping, fists clenched, lips trembling, eyes downcast or averted, cheeks pale or flushed, shoulders hunched or feet shuffling: these are all indications of John's feelings. What is more, the counsellor has to remember that this works both ways and that John is looking at him: John is liable to interpret the counsellor's behaviour too. If the counsellor is looking out of the window, rustling through files, yawning or coughing, taking notes assiduously, watching the clock, looking glazed or doodling, John may well think the counsellor is bored or disinterested in what he is saying. 'Just listening' requires great discipline and concentration on the part of the counsellor. The wise counsellor does not take on too many clients in too short a time, and gives himself time to breathe, think and relax between each interview in order not to succumb to fatigue.

One important problem counsellors have to face is how to be empathic, to show non-possessive warmth without becoming over-involved with their clients. However detached and professional the counsellor thinks he is, he is bound to be involved with John to an extent. Whether he likes it or not his personality and own attitudes are bound to be having an effect on John. It seems to me that there must be involvement between John and the counsellor for anything to happen at all. Paul Halmos discusses this point to great effect in *The Faith of the Counsellors.*[11] The danger point is reached when the counsellor is meeting his own needs through the interview as well as, or instead of, John's. When the counsellor himself feels angry with John's mother or the staff, and John, sensing this, thinks of the counsellor as an ally against the rest instead of someone who understands the point of view of both camps, then the counsellor becomes an alienator rather than a communicator. If the counsellor's own pride or need for success or results is at stake, then he risks pushing John into a solution which John does not accept for himself and which ultimately does not work for this reason. The counsellor is inevitably involved with the client but in a disciplined, professional way. Of course counsellors have needs: they may need to protect or to dominate, to be liked, to be systematic and orderly, or to be needed. It is to be hoped however that the counsellor's personal needs will be met primarily in his own private life, and such needs as do overspill into the counselling situation will be recognized by him and kept under his control. Clearly this is no easy task, which is one reason why counsellors themselves need regular discussion of their work. (The question of who shall counsel the counsellor will be taken up again in chapter 10.) Listening without interrupting, without leaping to conclusions, without leading the discussion away from what John really wants to talk about is difficult, and may be particularly difficult for someone who has taught and is used to a more dominant and active role. An inexperienced, nervous or anxious counsellor may find himself doing most of the talking: asking questions instead of letting John talk, filling in embarrassing silences with a change of subject, asking for information when what he really wants to hear about is John's feelings. John himself may avoid those topics that are painful to him initially, but he is more likely to talk about them if he is allowed to come to them in his own time and is not pressed when he needs silences to formulate what is so difficult to express.

The counsellor's first task is to let John talk, to let John feel that he is accepted and respected, to establish a relationship. He has to try to understand what John is saying, to see John and the people in John's life as John sees them, not as he himself would see them. He may need to restate to John what he thinks John has said in order to check this. Initially he is not concerned with the external truth so much as John's view of the world. He has to resist explaining to John prematurely what he thinks are the mechanisms of John's behaviour: for a start he may be wrong, particularly if he does this too soon, and in any case John may be more usefully helped to work this out for himself over a period of time. Interpretation may be frightening and unacceptable to John, and only cause him to block even more the path to the truth.

During the interview, the counsellor has very little time to work out what is happening, and often it is only in retrospect that he and perhaps John can begin to see what it was all about. Listening to a tape-recording of an interview can be a rewarding way of improving counselling techniques though this can only be done if the client agrees and is not inhibited by the presence of a machine. Otherwise writing a verbatim account of an interview can help a counsellor to perceive his most glaring technical defects and to understand what has happened.

What does counselling achieve?

We have discussed some of the qualities in a counselling relationship and we have said so far that the role of the counsellor is to get John to talk about his feelings and his problems with the aim of achieving greater self-understanding and self-acceptance. What happens next? What effect does this have on John? Sceptics might say that all John has learnt is to talk about his problems, and that this in itself is not going to alter John's problems or his behaviour in any way. But the point is that John's problems and John's social situation may be unalterable, and perhaps the only factor that can be altered is John's perception of his situation, which may be distorted. John's behaviour cannot begin to take a turn for the better until he understands the stresses in his life and becomes confident enough to be able to tolerate them. Then he may well begin to try out new patterns of behaviour, to make decisions, to take action on his own behalf. In this sense counselling may facilitate the learning of new behaviour patterns. But first the *mens sana* may need extra attention to achieve the balanced, tolerant view of life necessary for constructive and purposeful action and experiment. Those of us who have taught know from our own experience that some children *will* improve if they are exhorted or threatened, punished or rewarded. We may get results this way, though we should question how much these methods help our charges to grow up, to mature, to become responsible. But there are certainly other pupils who respond to none of these approaches. These children above all may need the particular kind of attention, the completely different kind of approach which the counsellor can provide because of his special role.

How can the counsellor establish a normal healthy 'preventive' service which is accepted and used spontaneously by pupils? It is not an easy task. Young people are unlikely to turn to someone they do not know at all: they only have the counsellor's word for it that he is trustworthy and respects confidences, and they mostly need more reassurance than that. If the counsellor teaches as well as counsels, he will be better known; he will have been tested out in the classroom situation and assessed by his charges. But the teacher/counsellor runs the risk of being perceived as an instrument of authority by the pupils and himself feeling conflict between his two roles. If he is nevertheless successful to an extent, he may well find his colleagues jealous of his achievements. The issue of whether counsellors should teach as well is one which provokes intense debate in the teaching profession and convincing arguments on either side. If we accept that the counsellor should not teach, then we have to think of a way for the counsellor to make contact with all the pupils, to be able to explain the nature and purpose of his service, to show that it is both normal and healthy to need and use such a service at times, to be tested out and assessed by the pupils. It is not enough for the counsellor to address a year or even a form and tell them why he is there: most of what he says will not be taken in and may leave the impression that his service is somehow abnormal. Once he is really established, word will get round as to how he operates and how trustworthy or helpful he is. But until that point, what can he do to establish rapport and trust with his future clients?

One way of doing this is for the counsellor to run a series of group discussions on human relationships. This is something we tried out. As a result of these discussion groups, about a third of the pupils came for counselling of their own accord at some stage during their school career. In the next chapter I propose to describe in detail how the scheme works.

References

1. L. Tyler *The Work of the Counselor*(Appleton Century Crofts 1961)
2. E. Erickson *Identity: Youth and Crisis* (Faber and Faber 1968)
3. B. Stefflre (ed) *Theories of Counseling* (McGraw-Hill 1965)

4. J. Warters *Techniques of Counseling* (McGraw-Hill 1964)
5. C. Rogers *Client-centered Therapy* (Houghton Mifflin 1951)
6. C. Rogers *On Becoming a Person* (Houghton Mifflin 1961)
7. E. Williamson *Counseling Adolescents* (McGraw-Hill 1950)
8. S. Hamrin and B. Paulson *Counseling Adolescents* (Science Research Associates 1950)
9. A. Boy and G. Pine *Client-centered Counseling in the Secondary School* (Houghton Mifflin 1963)
10. J. Krumboltz (ed) *Revolution in Counseling* (Houghton Mifflin 1966)
11. P. Halmos *The Faith of the Counsellors* (Constable 1965)

Chapter 4

Establishing a counselling service in a secondary school

The basic framework of the counselling scheme we devised is simple. It is designed to encourage self-referrals as much as possible; by this I mean that the students themselves come voluntarily and spontaneously for help when they think they need help. Obviously teaching staff suggest to certain girls that they might like to come for counselling, but they are never forced to see the counsellor. Because of this emphasis, the counsellors do not help every girl who needs help, only those who want help. Effective counselling at any level depends upon the co-operation of the client. Giving the girls themselves the responsibility and the opportunity of deciding whether to come for counselling helps to ensure this co-operation.

Part of the problem for the counsellor is to define realistic aims which are within the limits of his capabilities and, furthermore, to learn to use constructively the resources of his colleagues on the staff, and within the community welfare services. His role is not at all defined, and different counsellors may evolve different but equally valid schemes, all of which will have certain advantages and certain limitations.

In this chapter I want to describe the particular scheme of counselling which evolved over a period of time in the girls' comprehensive school where I worked. There were at that time two part-time counsellors on the staff. We each took specific responsibility for half the girls in the school, ie 1000 each, but in fact we concentrated our main efforts on the third year girls, who were all given an opportunity to talk to us. Of the 180 third year girls assigned to each counsellor, only about 20 per annum were counselled in any depth, though many others came once or twice. Thus the actual, as opposed to the potential, caseload of each counsellor was not very large. I offer our scheme for critical scrutiny in the belief that some parts of it will be useful, other parts may be discarded or improved, but that most of it will be of interest as an early working model.

It seems important, to give our scheme any coherence, to begin by explaining something of the organization of the school at that time, the reasons why counselling was introduced, and how and why the counselling scheme was devised.

The organization of the school

The school itself is a large comprehensive for girls in an urban area. It is fortunate in that it *is* comprehensive in three ways: socio-economic, intellectual and cultural. It contains a healthy mixture of girls with widely different social backgrounds and of various nationalities, and there is a balanced intake of intellectual ability, with no shortage of highly intelligent girls. In other words it is not a school which draws on one housing estate or one stratum of society, and it is not intellectually impoverished.

The school is unstreamed, with a 12 form entry, that is, 360 girls in each academic year. Each form of 30 girls is put in the charge of a form tutor who is responsible for their pastoral care. Her role is clearly specified by the head; the phrase 'form tutor' rather than 'form teacher' is used to denote the extent of her responsibility for each individual. The form tutor stays with her form for at least three years. The 12 form tutors in each year are in turn responsible to the year mistress who looks after the 360 girls in her charge throughout their school career. The deputy head concerns herself especially with the third and fourth years, the head with all the other years. Thus there is a continuity of care and consistency of concern for each individual girl. The children have a great sense of belonging both to their tutor group and their year; this identification with a small group provides for the children a stable and secure home base which is both a refuge and a strength to them. The children very often confide in their tutors, and the tutors themselves talk over their problems with the senior staff.

The system of pastoral care is therefore, as in most schools, carefully thought out and actively used. The fact that the head and the staff decided this was not enough is in itself testimony to their sensitivity and deep concern in this field. They felt that in addition there was a place for someone to *supplement* the work of the form tutor. The form tutors recognized that they did not have time amidst their many other duties to give sufficient attention to the few girls in each form with serious problems. They also recognized that some children might want to talk to someone outside the structure of the school system, someone who would listen but who would not be bound by virtue of her office to take disciplinary action. This is not to say that girls do not confide in their form tutor; some do and some confide in a subject teacher but just a few need the reassurance of someone who can be trusted with confidential information, who is outside the disciplinary role.

It was important that the head and staff themselves thought of the idea originally, and really wanted a counsellor. Pioneering any new job is no easy task, but the task was made simpler because of the co-operation and support of the head and her staff. Goodwill, acceptance and positive regard from colleagues are as important to the work of the counsellor as to any individual. Staff attitudes to counselling are readily conveyed to pupils and had they been negative could easily have undermined the system. It is not every teacher who can easily share her children and bear not to know everything about them; yet this ability to let go the child to the counsellor, in the ultimate interest of the child, was one of the most helpful staff characteristics.

Aims and principles

When we first began to discuss our scheme in October 1964 we thought of counselling as a way of promoting positive mental health. The head herself had taken an active part in a conference on this subject organized by the National Association for Mental Health in 1963 and I had recently completed training as a Marriage Guidance Education Counsellor. We found that we had similar objectives in mind, all of which are concerned with mental health:

(1) to help individuals through temporary crises
(2) to help adolescents with normal developmental problems
(3) to note signs of abnormal disturbance at the earliest stages
(4) to refer cases needing specialist treatment at the earliest possible opportunity
(5) to help communications within and between the school, the home, the community and its resources
(6) to support teachers who are helping individuals in their care but who themselves want reassurance and guidance.

Before we actually began our counselling experiment in September 1965 several further important points were established. These were the principles of confidentiality, availability and acceptability.

Confidentiality has already been discussed in chapter 3. A client-centred service can be on no other basis but that of absolute trust between counsellor and pupil. For the counsellor to reveal what is confidential is not only unethical, but also completely undermines the service provided. The counsellor's reputation for trustworthiness or otherwise will have serious repercussions on the effectiveness of the counselling service. Confidentiality is sometimes hard for teaching colleagues to accept, yet it is possible for a counsellor to communicate with them in general terms and in a positive way without breaking confidentiality; it is however *impossible* for a counsellor to help her clients to express their feelings fully if they are not confident of her integrity.

Availability. The principle of availability is linked closely with the idea of encouraging self-referrals rather than staff-referrals. Most counselling interviews have to be arranged with an official appointment: this seems essential for smooth administration, also less disruptive for classes and less irritating for teachers. The form tutor hands out an appointment slip which serves as an official pass for leaving a particular lesson to come for counselling. But because we feared certain girls might be put off by this official red tape, we have always made it clear that the counsellor can be contacted directly in her room, before or after school or between lessons. Problems do not fit neatly into timetables; good communication with the counsellor demands that she should be accessible. She cannot however take on every client who knocks on her door, there and then. An acute crisis may not be the best moment to begin constructive counselling: the form teacher may have to bear the brunt of the emotional outburst while the counsellor reassures the child that she can have an appointment in the near future. When the emotional storm has passed, the child may be in a better position to look at its underlying causes.

Acceptability. To begin to function at all adequately the counsellor has to be accepted not only by the pupils but also by the staff, parents and social welfare agencies. Gaining acceptance from all these groups takes time. We had to begin with the immediate environment. We set up discussion groups to gain acceptance from our potential clients, the girls. To gain acceptance from the staff, we had to make it clear that the counsellor's role was *different* from the form tutors' and that the counsellor was in no way taking over the year mistresses' or form tutors' responsibility for the pupils but that she was simply a supplementary benefit providing an ancillary service of a completely different kind. *How* we made this clear is a subject which I shall take up again in chapter 5.

Role limitations

From the beginning we set certain limitations on the counsellor's role: she would not teach; she would not undertake vocational guidance, educational guidance or psychological testing. Our reasons for making these decisions were simple and practical.

No teaching

The counsellor would not teach because she would not have time to teach; to do so would take her away from her main purpose, counselling. She would not have time to teach because she was going to begin, experimentally, on a part-time basis. Even if she had time to teach, there was the possibility of this causing confusion about her role both for herself and for the pupils. In a school as large as ours the teaching role would not particularly help the counsellor to know her clients in their normal setting, for she would only be able to teach a small proportion of them. In any case it is arguable whether it is a good idea for the counsellor to risk prejudicing her view of the child through classroom experience. Because of her peripheral role, the counsellor walks a delicate tightrope across many boundaries. There is some respite for the counsellor in not having to face the additional conflict of the dual role of teacher/counsellor. There are disadvantages too. For example the counsellor has relatively little light relief and may get out of touch with normality. For the girls in our school however we were able to define the counsellor's role as different from the teacher's role. Thus the counsellor is accepted by the teaching staff as a colleague, which is essential, yet in the girls' eyes is perceived as someone standing slightly apart from the school 'system'. This has made it easier for the girls to talk, in confidence, about problems which they imagine might affront or worry unduly someone in a position of authority. The counsellor is not 'agin the government': this would make her a destructive and damaging force within the school. But she does not feel for example that she must enforce school regulations at all costs. *Not* teaching helps to free her from this kind of subtle pressure within herself to enforce conformity.

No vocational guidance

In the school there are two careers mistresses. The careers room is open daily before and after school. The careers officers of the local careers office come into the school from the third year onwards. Much is done to help the girls make wise vocational decisions. Deciding that the counsellor should not provide vocational guidance did not mean that we felt no more could be done in this field. It meant that we recognized that if the counsellor undertook vocational guidance she would probably have little time left for the personal problems which may well lie at the base of a vocational problem; vocational guidance is easier and more effective when the client is free from emotional strain and conflict. Furthermore whilst vocational guidance is easier and more effective when the client is free from emotional strain and conflict. Furthermore whilst problems before they reach the careers officer, it is also a highly skilled and specialized job in a technical sense. It requires considerable knowledge not only of job qualifications and conditions but of developing national manpower trends and local fluctuations in job opportunities. In other words, we respected the careers officers' specialized training and skills for providing this kind of service, and recognized that our role was not to compete with their expertise but to be supportive to it. It is true that there is a case for having more vocational guidance in schools; but the counsellor who undertakes this has to recognize that the burden of paper work and administration which may accrue as a result may prevent his having time for or even perceiving the extent of the fundamental personal problems of his clients. The counsellor must decide what he is most able to do and apportion his time accordingly. In our case we decided that the counsellor would refer to the careers teacher or careers officer any cases needing vocational guidance.

No educational guidance

We also decided that the counsellor should not undertake educational guidance for similar reasons: an effective system of guidance already existed; to undertake educational guidance would be time-consuming and might divert the counsellor from clients' more basic problems; the year mistresses and form tutors, guided by the head and deputy head, were in a better position than the counsellor to help pupils with their choices of subject and course, because they have a more balanced overall view of the individual's work, progress and behaviour over a period of time. Because of her non-teaching role, the counsellor would be at a disadvantage in assessing pupils' abilities realistically. Where completely objective assessment of a pupil's abilities was required, then the educational psychologist could be asked to administer appropriate tests. The range of choice in the middle school is limited compared with that in an American high school. One of the aims of the school is to keep individuals' options open as long as possible by providing a curriculum which is as open-ended as possible within the confines and restrictions of the further education system and the needs of those who really do want to take specialized vocational courses while still at school. The decision we made then was that the counsellor was not necessarily the person best suited to provide educational guidance and that her limited time and talents were more urgently needed elsewhere—namely in the realm of personal problems.

The role of the counsellor *vis-à-vis* the child guidance clinic had to be worked out most carefully. The existing system was that referrals to the child guidance clinic could in obvious cases be made direct by the school with parental agreement, or by parents. More often the educational psychologist attached to the local child guidance clinic who visits the school regularly would be asked to assess, sometimes to test, children about whom the staff were worried and to make recommendations for action where appropriate. The educational psychologist continued to be used by the school exactly as before: staff refer to her directly and occupy her time fully. What the counselling service does is to provide another source of referral, based on what the girls feel about themselves. For what is interesting and disturbing about the system of self-referrals we have established is the number of serious problems which have come to light which otherwise might have gone undetected and unsolved. These are, in particular, girls whose work and behaviour are not remarkable in any way, who may be functioning in school quite adequately, yet who in fact have serious problems. 'She could do better': this category of girl may be covering up a mild depression or difficult social situation. This may be *why* she is not giving her best.

Counsellors do not replace educational psychologists: they need them for advice and guidance. They in turn support the work of the school psychological services by helping with early detection and referral of serious problems. We have found the existence of a counselling service has improved, not undermined, the relationship between the school and the child guidance clinic. We have found the support of the school psychological services essential to the proper functioning of our work. Chapter 9 will discuss in more detail how we organize communication, co-operation and case discussion with this and other vital ancillary social welfare services. For the moment the point I want to make clear is that we defined the work of the counsellor as closely allied to that of the psychological and welfare services but to do with a different category of children. Our work was to be with 'normal' children, in the broadest sense, theirs with children needing more highly specialized treatment. We know that there is no such thing as 'normal'. What we mean by this loose term is simply that our province is children who do not need any kind of special education or medical or psychiatric treatment; children who are being educated in the environment most appropriate for their age, ability and aptitude but who need some supportive counselling at times to give them the assurance and peace of mind necessary for full development of their potential. When we discover a child with problems needing more specialized or expert attention than we can provide, then we make referrals; at all times we consult the experts to make sure that we are not trying to carry or sustain problems which we are not able to help constructively. If for any reason (such as parental refusal) we are not able to bring in the specialist help required, then we ourselves consult the specialists for guidance.

Reaching our clients

Having established that the counsellor would not undertake teaching, psychological testing, vocational or educational guidance, but would concentrate on the personal problems of the normal individual, we had to think of a way for the counsellor to reach these individuals. One possibility was for the counsellor to sit in her room, labelled *Advice Centre*, and to wait for customers to come. We felt that whereas in the community setting this kind of approach can be fruitful (as for example in the consultation centres at Hampstead, Brent, Notting Hill, Bristol etc) in the school setting all but the most extrovert might be daunted initially, until the service had been proven. It would be difficult to communicate the aims and frame of reference of the service; an assembly of pupils addressed by the counsellor might have some effect but we felt that even this would leave the majority of the pupils sceptical and confused about the nature, the value and the trustworthiness of the service. This approach was too passive; the 'ever open door' and the mass communication meeting could be tried and were tried but were not enough in themselves.

Another way of reaching clients might be for form tutors to refer to the counsellor, girls who were causing them some concern. There are two objections to this scheme: first there is a danger that the counsellor may be used by the form teacher as a punishment or threat. The girl may see the counsellor as just another arm of the law and refuse to co-operate. An experienced counsellor will be aware of the dangers of manipulation by pupil or teacher; a skilled counsellor may be able to overcome any initial hostility or misapprehension in the client. But in certain cases the co-operation of the client will not be forthcoming, which makes counselling impossible. Second the children who are causing the form teacher most concern are not necessarily the ones needing the most extra attention. Law breakers, window breakers, paper throwers, rabble rousers are easy enough to spot; so are teachers' pets, complete isolates, weepers and wailers. Even some of these categories of difficult child are sometimes not brought to the attention of authority until more than one teacher is suffering at their hands, and the problem in no way discredits the ability of the teacher to control a class. Given that even the most obvious problem children may not be helped in the earliest stages of their difficulties, because of the teacher's fear of appearing or being inadequate, we have to face the further point that some problems are not obvious. Children may be labouring under quite serious stresses and strains which for personal reasons they may cover up in public. Form teachers may be aware of this of course but it cannot be assumed *automatically* that the form teacher's judgement of which children need counselling will tally absolutely with the children's actual needs. It is highly likely that the form teacher's judgement will be right but this cannot be assumed. It is rather like asking a teacher to send forward for X-ray only the children she thinks might have TB. If a screening service is to be reliable, everyone must be screened. The advantage of the counsellor's seeing everyone is that the children have the opportunity of expressing their difficulties, if any, for themselves. When they do this they are in effect asking the counsellor for help, which means that she may be able to help them. If she unearths problems she cannot help, at least she is able to bring in the appropriate specialist.

This brings us to the consideration of a scheme in which the counsellor simply interviews everybody. If the counsellor's reputation is already established, and if he is equipped with extraordinary personal qualities, or a good screening tool (ie a test for picking out potentially disturbed children), this method could achieve good results. We rejected it because we felt that it was too inquisitorial and that girls might not respond to sudden questioning by a complete stranger even though the stranger reassured them with promises of confidentiality. Psychiatric screening based on a few key questions might well be something to combine with a school medical, conducted in the presence of and with the agreement of the parent: the ethic of the medical profession is generally understood and patients are used to being asked personal questions by doctors and giving routine answers to them. We felt that the role and ethic of the counsellor was not then sufficiently understood or accepted to justify systematic questioning: we felt that girls and parents might object, and might object with reason, to being asked questions about their private lives by a counsellor. If pupils or parents tell us voluntarily about their problems, this is a completely different matter.

Any other objection to the routine question and answer interview is the effect it might have on any potential counselling relationship. Apart from the suspicion or hostility which might be aroused in the client, it also puts the counsellor, from the very beginning, in a judgemental, expert role. Administering a questionnaire is an impersonal objective activity which avoids the necessity of making a relationship: it is a less strenuous activity for the counsellor but it does not promote the formation of a relationship which is so essential to counselling itself. Asking questions in a friendly chat is a more personalized way of getting information but is liable not to elicit the whole truth because it is unlikely that any bond of trust and confidence will be established with the counsellor in a few minutes, except in a minority of cases. Someone who has come forward for counselling does not mind giving information, but this is because she has already demonstrated this intention and her good faith by seeking an interview.

So whilst we accepted that it was important for the counsellor to interview every child at some stage during her school career, we felt that the value of the interview could be enhanced if the counsellor already knew all the pupils well enough for them to trust her and to *want* to confide in her. Teaching an ordinary school subject would bring the counsellor in touch with only a few pupils. Teaching religious education might be another way of making brief contact with a large number of pupils, though the religious education teacher has to spread himself throughout so many classes for so few periods a week that he may find he has little opportunity of getting to know his pupils individually; he will in any case probably be regarded, whatever he is really like, as being a staunch supporter of law and order and a maintainer of the *status quo*. He has an important role to play in a school: but because of his association with religion, pupils in fact may not express their true feelings to him as much as he may think.

Thus although religious education teaching could be a way for the counsellor to make contact with pupils, an even freer and less authority-loaded approach might be through discussions on human relationships. This we decided would be our way of making contact with pupils, explaining our role, being tested out by the pupils and beginning to establish the rapport which could form the basis of a counselling relationship later, if necessary. This approach most satisfied our aim of establishing a service which was neither too passive nor obtrusive upon personal liberty, a service which gave an equal chance for every individual to ask for help if and when she should need it. It was no accident that we decided to use group discussion of human relationships in this way, for two reasons. Both myself and my colleague, who joined me a term after I began, were trained as Marriage Guidance Education Counsellors. It was this training which helped us more than anything else to formulate the conceptual frame of reference upon which our experiment was based and which led us naturally to think of group work with children as a way of making contact with them and explaining our role. The second reason we began in this way was that the school already used outside speakers for discussion groups about human relationships with the third year girls.

From our experience of taking similar discussions in schools, on behalf of the Marriage Guidance Council, we knew that often girls would come up afterwards with a pressing personal problem. Because we were 'just visiting' we were unable to help them in any sustained way. Being permanently attached to a school meant that our group work could be more thorough because we would have more sessions with smaller groups, and that we would be able to give a series of counselling interviews for those who asked for help and for as long as they wished. Furthermore these would be self-referrals which we regarded as of fundamental importance to the working of the scheme.

Taking over and extending something already established made our scheme immediately more acceptable and comprehensible to staff and students; the fact that previously it had been thought necessary to use outside speakers in this role, to allow absolute freedom of discussion, helped us to preserve the role of outsider—a role which has frustrating limitations at times but which certainly encourages girls, individually and in groups, to speak freely.

The structuring of the groups

In deciding to continue the discussions already established with the third year girls (aged 13-14) we bore in mind the following considerations. Some girls are ready for this sort of discussion before the third year, others not till later, but by and large this is the year when the onset of puberty brings in its wake a whole host of developmental problems, many of which manifest themselves in difficult behaviour. The little girl of yesteryear may suddenly become a demonic siren, fluctuating between insolent independence and desperate dependence. She does not know how to handle her new self and quite often neither do we. But she is certainly growing conscious of her own sexuality and glad to join in discussions which deal not just with the facts of life, which have already been covered in human biology, but with her own feelings, her hopes and fears, her illusions and her expectations. Her problems may not be primarily how to deal with the opposite sex, so much as how to gain her independence and what to do with it when she has it. Growing up physically brings with it a whole new set of difficulties in learning how to relate to people: at home, at school, with the opposite sex and in society. This is what our group discussions are really all about.

In the third year of the school there are 12 forms, each containing about 30 girls aged 13-14 years. Six forms (that is about 180 girls) are allocated to each of the two counsellors, who then takes responsibility for these particular girls throughout their school life. As the academic year divides into six half terms, each counsellor devotes half a term to concentrated work with each of the six forms for whom she is responsible. We spend the first three weeks of the half term in group discussions, sometimes taking a double session, sometimes taking one morning and one afternoon session of the same day. The second three weeks are for individual counselling. In all, the form misses six lessons to come to the discussions. Which lessons they miss is worked out carefully with the staff, who mostly recognize that this is not an insuperable blow to their syllabus and may reap rewards in other ways.

We do not see the whole of each form at a time: there are approximately 30 girls in each form and this is too many for an effective group discussion in which all members can feel sufficiently free and confident to participate. Each form is therefore divided into two groups of 15; even this is rather too many and three groups of 10 might be better. But with limited time at our disposal we had to make a practical decision: to do the group work more thoroughly would leave even less time for work with individuals. This way we also disrupt fewer lessons, probably to the relief of the teaching staff. At least it can be argued that our discussions do not take up a disproportionate amount of time or get adolescent problems out of perspective.

The division into groups

We do not divide the girls into their groups of 15: the girls divide *themselves*, by a simple sociometric technique. Just before the group work is to begin, the form teacher explains something of what the discussions over the next few weeks will be about and what a counsellor is. She then picks out two girls, both popular, but quite different kinds of girls; she may choose Mary, who represents the quieter, 'sensible' element in the form, and Marilyn, who represents the boisterous, 'sexy' set. Both girls may be mature, or maturing fast, but in different ways. The rest of the form then decide for themselves which group they want to join.

We have found by experimenting that this method has certain advantages over the teacher's own groupings. The teacher can judge physical and social maturity, but the other important factor to take into account is the natural groupings of friends, the social networks in each form. There will probably be more than two natural groups in each form, but provided they understand something of the nature of the groups, the girls are very good judges of where they belong. Of the two resultant groups, one may be marginally more mature, more blatantly 'sexy', but both will be based on an existing network of relationships, which greatly helps the cohesiveness of the groups. The girls are more relaxed, more able to bring out their real feelings among people they know and trust already. Just occasionally we are faced with one wild, garrulous group, and one passive inarticulate group, but more normally there is a developmental spread in each group. We certainly prefer this to a group divided alphabetically or completely randomly by the form tutor. Our self-selection method avoids also a feeling that the groups have been graded into the haves and the have nots, which is certainly not the intention but which has been expressed by groups chosen by the form teacher. Our self-selection method not only brings us a more cohesive group, but demonstrates from the very beginning our willingness to let adolescents take responsibility for themselves.

The physical structuring of the groups

We do not have counselling rooms specifically and permanently set aside for our use. We borrow rooms from other departments for our exclusive use on the days we are in school. Thus the girls know where to find us when they want to come for individual counselling. If they have an urgent problem they know that they can catch us to make an appointment in our rooms between lessons, or before or after school. The rooms are not specially or luxuriously appointed, and this is of no great importance. What is important is that they are not cluttered with rows of desks, they are small, they are not overlooked by passers-by: this helps to ensure a degree of informality, privacy and security. The girls sit in a circle of chairs, without desks, and the counsellor is a part of this circle.

The physical structure of the group is important. By making herself a part of the circle, instead of being ensconced on a throne or dais, or installed behind a desk, the counsellor diminishes to an extent the tendency the group may have to regard her as the leader and the expert. The discussions are then more likely to be centred on the needs of the group and less dominated by the counsellor. The circular structure ensures that every member has an equal chance of participating, of seeing everybody; of being involved, and that nobody is, by some quirk of fate, forced to take a back seat, allowed to hide behind someone else or put into a dominant position which upsets the balance of the group.

In the first group discussion it is vital for the counsellor to explain her job, her role, her way of working; she tells the group that in all they will meet six times during the next three weeks and that after that they will be able to come for individual counselling if they so wish. She explains about confidentiality, she encourages the group to express what they really feel rather than what they think they ought to feel, reassuring them that the contents of the discussion will not be passed on to the staff or their parents; and that the counsellor herself will not mind what is said, that no subject is taboo if this is what the group really wants to discuss. The group will probably not believe this at first; the counsellor will probably find that the group brings up some sensational 'shocking' subjects in order to test this out. If the counsellor survives this, the group will then begin to have sufficient confidence in her to talk more normally about their real problems.

What actually goes on in the group discussions is such a fascinating and vast topic that to discuss it in detail now would divert me from my present task which is to lay bare the bones of our scheme. I shall come back to the content of the group discussions later on when I discuss adolescent problems. All I want to do now is to make a few points about the group discussions. It does not really matter what the girls discuss in the group. There is no syllabus and there are very few 'red herrings' because the aim of the group discussion is not to put across certain information but to allow the girls to talk about their feelings. 'Red herrings' may occur when one girl dominates the group with a long personal story which may act as a damper to the expression of feelings by others, when the group is too dependent on the counsellor or when two particular girls take up a dialogue to the exclusion of all others. But these are not blockages of subject matter so much as blockages of psychological mechanism.

We must distinguish between the kind of group work undertaken by counsellors and that sometimes undertaken by teachers. A skilful teacher may manipulate a group to argue out a case and to come to a logical conclusion; but it is the conclusion that the teacher has wanted the group to reach—the 'right' answer, based on facts. He has not put words into people's mouths, but he has asked the right questions at the right times. This technique of innocent ignorance is a valuable teaching tool. 'But why do you think he did that?' 'How did it get there in the first place?' In group counselling this technique has little place. The counsellor is not manipulating the group for his own end, to make them believe 'the facts', because he is not dealing with facts but with feelings and these are necessarily subjective and individual. The teacher who leads group counselling discussions must therefore be prepared to allow discussion which may go against his own views; he must be prepared *not* to come in at the end—*deus ex machina*—with the right answer. He must have a view but he must be able to tolerate that not everybody need share it. The teacher in the classroom can air his views without necessarily having them questioned and an uncomfortable challenger can soon be cut down to size with sleight of tongue. The counsellor cannot do this if the group is to be at all free.

Given that we spend at most two out of six sessions answering and discussing questions to do with love, sex, sexual behaviour and related social problems, it must be evident that these topics are given relatively scant treatment. It would be possible to spend an academic term or year discussing each and every issue properly. Many of the topics raised in our groups, such as the meaning of love, the purpose of marriage, abortion, homosexuality, are brought up in discussion in the teaching of other subjects: human biology, religious knowledge and English in particular. We think it important that the whole staff should be involved in this, as indeed they are, and we value the spontaneous discussion which arises from the study of a set text or the debate of a moral principle in lessons. But the purposes of these discussions may be different from ours. Our discussions are to give the girls the opportunity to discuss freely those few things they might feel unable to ask their parents or their form teacher; to help them not to be afraid to communicate their feelings to adults; to lay the foundations of a relationship between them and the counsellor to the end that they will feel sufficient confidence in the counsellor to come for help when they need it; to give the girls an opportunity of testing out the counsellor, of deciding whether they like and trust her; to give the counsellor an opportunity of seeing how a girl behaves in her peer group.

This last point is important for the non-teaching counsellor; the group work provides her with a brief glimpse of the way the girls relate to each other. It is doubtful whether a teacher/counsellor would teach everybody who came for counselling, and so for him too, group work could be useful. A counsellor who has taken a group six times is not going to have anywhere near such an accurate picture of the child's general behaviour as the counsellor who has taught a child for a year or so. But then, if the counsellor is trying to see the world as the client sees it, he is likely to find this easier if his view is not prejudiced by the classroom experience: if Joan is the ringleader of the group which undermines your lessons, it is difficult to help her as objectively as you would wish. The counsellor in the group discussions has the advantage of not needing to enforce discipline, rules or punishment and this makes it easier to view the group, however many troublemakers it contains, with a certain objective benevolence. But he can notice certain things about individuals in the group. In our groups we might notice that Mary never says a word, and does not appear to have a mate. We might observe that June needs to be dominant in the group, that Molly gets very emotional in discussion, that Kate opts out and that Pat always tries to sit next to the counsellor. There may not be very much significance in these observations: type-casting by the counsellor on such flimsy evidence could be damaging and misleading. But we bear our observations in mind when we see the girls individually.

The autobiographical note

Every girl in the third year, then, is seen by one or other of the counsellors for six discussions about human relationships. In the fourth or fifth discussion group, we ask the girls to write an unstructured autobiographical note. We explain carefully that the purpose of the note is to enable the counsellor to get to know them in order to be able to help them if and when necessary. We stress that the note is for our own use and will not be shown to their teachers or parents without the individual's permission. We say that they can tell us as much or as little as they like about themselves and their families. Our reasons for this permissive approach are these: we know that some families resent any intrusion into their private lives and we respect this right to keep one's private life private. For example, a girl may want to keep secret from everybody, including us, the fact that her parents are separated, possibly because this is the wish of her parents.

We ask the girls to tell us, if they want to, something about their parents, their brothers and sisters (with ages), the way they spend their spare time, what they want to do when they leave school and anything else they think would interest us and help us to get to know and understand them. This last open-ended clause is one which often brings, much to our surprise, the written expression of a serious problem. More normally, the note is relatively guarded and the problem, if any, is left to the face-to-face interviews. A few girls express their feelings more easily on paper than verbally but this is not usually the case. When we first began doing this we asked for the autobiographical note in the second or third meeting. Later we changed this to the fourth or fifth. The difference in the kind of remarks made was amazing. Clearly even by the second or third session the girls are not sure how much they trust the counsellor. By the time they get to the fourth or fifth session, and assuming they are ever going to trust the counsellor, they are feeling more certain.

The autobiographical notes provide a wealth of illuminating comments on life which I propose to discuss later. For the moment all I want to say is that the autobiographical note is *not* a reliable indicator of whether a girl needs further help. The quality of the note is greatly influenced by such factors as the girl's ability to write, and how reserved she is generally. Some girls are guarded in what they write and understandably so. Some notes are surprisingly emotional and dramatic and the counsellor has to be careful not to read too much into them. Because the note is voluntary there is no knowing whether information, significant or insignificant, has been suppressed or concealed, distorted, exaggerated or simply omitted. Were we trying to get a systematic factual picture of the background of each girl, we should not allow them to write an unstructured note, we should administer a questionnaire. What we are interested in is not so much the facts of a girl's life, but the way she feels about people and things in her life. It therefore does not matter to us initially whether the girl is exaggerating, or how much she is hiding. This is something which will emerge if and when she comes for counselling interviews.

Having the autobiographical note in hand does however help the counsellors to remember which girl is which. Without them we should quickly forget the little we have gleaned about the girls in the six discussion groups. It gives us a peg on which to hang our own impressions of the girls; this is particularly important in discussions with staff. It also helps to refresh our memories when a girl returns for counselling spontaneously two or three years after she has been in our groups. The girl's emotional situation may have completely changed by then but it is obviously more encouraging and reassuring to the child if the counsellor remembers something about her life. Even if the counsellor does not remember her particularly well the girl feels that the counsellor knows her and cares about her, and this attitude facilitates the establishment of a counselling relationship.

The standard interview

In the last of the six sessions with the counsellor every member of the group is interviewed briefly. The purpose of the interview is to establish whether the child wants to come for further counselling. Each child is given an equal chance of stating this in private. We do not ask those who want to come for further counselling to put up their hands or sign a list. We feel that not only would this contradict our aim of showing respect for each individual child, but that it would also not bring us the right customers. The rowdy, unruly element in each form is not going to admit publicly that it wants help. The shy or withdrawn children may not feel sufficient confidence to show their needs in front of others. In the brief interview the child is not jumping on to a bandwagon—she is stating her preference without being sure what her friends are doing. While the interviews are being conducted the rest of the group discusses any remaining issues or finishes reading the books or the Marriage Guidance Council pamphlets which the counsellor has lent them.

Both counsellors are fortunate in having a room for discussion groups which is divided from the main thoroughfares by a small lobby. This lobby is useful both as a secluded waiting room for clients and also for this routine interview. At this stage there is only time for a short interview of five minutes or less. This is not the moment to begin counselling proper as there are too many pressures of time and too many people to see. There are few cases so urgent that they cannot wait for a proper appointment. Where a girl has stated in her autobiographical note that she has a problem, it is simply a case of reassuring her as to how soon an appointment for a counselling interview can be arranged. Some girls have given no indication of any problem either on paper or in the group, and most of these, after a few minutes' chat, say that there was nothing they wanted to talk over at greater length. They are reminded that they can always come back later if they change their minds: occasionally they do this.

Some girls write rather inadequate notes and the counsellor checks over details such as the ages of brothers and sisters. The counsellor might notice for example that there is no mention of dad, and will ask about him. If it turns out that he is dead, or is not living with his family for some reason, the counsellor will tread gently, giving the girl an opportunity to talk more, but at the same time trying not to reopen old wounds which may have healed over. What is missing in the autobiographical note can often be as important as what is expressed: but if a point is not mentioned precisely because it is a sore point, and a confidential one at that, the counsellor respects the girl's right to keep her family life to herself and does not press too hard. Some of the girls stand out from the way they have behaved in the group as being in need of extra care and attention, but not all the most hard-bitten young misses want to turn to the counsellor for help. We might give extra encouragement to those *we* think need our help to come for counselling but we certainly do not in any way force them to come, because we do not think we would be able to help them on these terms. We do not in any case normally undertake supportive work with girls who are already in care, on probation or seeing a psychiatrist unless we are asked to do so by the agency concerned. Quite a few girls slip through our net because of this permissive non-directive approach of ours but at least we *are* another net, and we do counsel a lot of girls whose needs have passed unnoticed up to that point.

Individual problems

My records show that in a form of 30 there are usually about 10 who ask for counselling. What kind of problems do they bring forward? Obviously there is no set pattern but we can give an approximate breakdown of numbers. Some six girls will have transitory developmental problems, particularly conflicts with parents about going out and having boyfriends. Two or three may have problems which are serious and disturbing but not to the extent of making their behaviour abnormal. These may be girls with home backgrounds which are genuinely difficult and hard to tolerate without support: marital disharmony, financial worries, overcrowding, aged grandparents, sibling rivalry, a handicapped brother or sister. One or two girls will have problems which are better referred to the child guidance clinic or social services. This is excluding those already benefiting from these special services. In particular many of the girls we find we can help are the 'could do betters'. They may not be much trouble, they may not be withdrawn or isolated, but they do need help if they are to do themselves justice. Merely stating that a child could do better does not help her to improve, and may even discourage her. If we feel a child could do better we need to ask why, and to try to get at the root cause.

We are well aware that it would be unrealistic to expect any one counsellor to suit the needs of every individual child. Some individuals may prefer to turn to some other member of staff when they need to talk or they may decide to keep their problems to themselves. In the groups the girls have had the opportunity to judge for themselves to what extent they think this particular counsellor is empathic, understanding, permissive, non-authoritarian, non-judgemental, trustworthy and genuine. On the basis of their assessment the girls decide whether to use the counselling service. Some never need to use the service and some never want to. Some do not need it just then, but they come back to the counsellor one, two or three years after the group discussions at a stage when they do want counselling. When girls who have been through our groups are referred to us later by staff, our task is again made easier.

The group work thus forms the basis of the relationship between the girl and the counsellor and increases thereafter the effectiveness of both self-referrals and staff-referrals because the role, aims, and methods of the counsellor are understood. They are understood not because the counsellor has explained them but because she is tested and known. Because it is normal for girls to come for counselling after the groups, going to see the counsellor does not become shameful or odd. Many girls go to see the counsellor and a child does not have to have 'terrible problems' to qualify. Girls who come for individual counselling do so in lesson time with an official appointment, and for as long as they wish. Most girls need to come only once or twice; but in each form there will be one or two at least who need regular counselling over a long period of time.

Chapter 5

Relationships between the school staff and the counsellors

What do the teachers think about counselling? How do the counsellors fit into the organization of the school? How do staff feel about letting girls out of lessons for group discussions and then, again, for individual counselling? The description of our counselling scheme would be incomplete without some explanation of how it fits into the organization of the school as a whole.

In describing the way we built up and worked out the teacher/counsellor relationship over a period of time, I shall attempt also to answer some of the many questions, both practical and personal, which counselling raises in teachers' minds. On the practical side, teachers whose pupils miss lessons to go for counselling are bound to ask whether the time is being wisely spent. Why not fit counselling into the lunch hour or after school? What effect does it have on a pupil's academic progress to miss parts of a syllabus? What effect does it have on lessons for pupils to go in and out? What effect does it have on the pupil to be singled out for counselling? Can the counsellor guarantee that this pupil will work better and learn more in future? Isn't the counsellor simply encouraging children to wallow in self-pity? What can the counsellor do, in such a short time, which is any better or any different from what everyone else has already tried? *Why* can't the counsellor sort out this problem (even though no one else has): what is the counsellor *for*? Is there not a danger that some pupils will just use the counsellor as another way of getting out of lessons?

On a personal level teachers may feel, though not very often voice, deeper anxieties. What is Jane saying about *them*? Is she criticizing them or their teaching methods? What will the counsellor do with this information? Supposing she believes it, supposing it is true, supposing she passes it on to the 'powers that be'?

These personal anxieties coupled with general scepticism about what counselling might achieve may lead to even more questions. *Why* won't the counsellor tell the staff about Jane's family's problems? How can the staff help her if they do not understand her background? Why is Jennifer going to see the counsellor? What is wrong with her? Who is this counsellor anyway?

One of the threads in the teacher's ambivalent feelings about the counsellor is the fear of being criticized by pupils. This fear is hardly ever expressed by staff, at a conscious level, yet it is a well justified fear, for girls very often *do* make criticisms of staff or the way the school is run, in the same way that they run down their parents. There may well therefore exist in a school which has a counsellor a feeling among the staff that the counsellor is loaded with a lot of damaging information which, although exaggerated and one-sided, might be used against a member of staff. Until teachers are able to see for themselves not only that this does not happen, but also that the counsellor does not hold grudges or anything else against them and that he respects and values them as individuals, then they are bound to have mixed feelings about him.

The head and his senior colleagues can clearly pave the way for the counsellor and without their support the counsellor is lost. But in the day-to-day work of the school, the quality of the actual teacher/counsellor relationship can subtly influence for better or for worse what the teacher is trying to do in the classroom and what the counsellor is trying to do in the counselling room.

It is therefore an important part of any counsellor's job to dispel any fears and misconceptions about himself; to define realistically, in as far as he is able, the limits and limitations of his job and himself; in other words, to form good relationships, to communicate his objectives, to create an atmosphere of trust and positive regard between himself and his colleagues. If he is not able to do this he should not be a counsellor. If he is anything of a counsellor, his colleagues will respond readily to this approach and give him the reassurance and co-operation he needs to function properly. His colleagues will respond even more sympathetically if he is prepared to admit his own doubts, worries and uncertainties from the beginning and share them.

Staff who are left in ignorance of what a counsellor is trying to do are not to be blamed if they react adversely. Those who imagine that the counsellor is a panacea for all ills will quickly be disappointed. Those who are inwardly resentful of the counsellor will seize triumphantly upon examples of what the counsellor is failing to achieve, not realizing that they are judging success solely from a teacher's viewpoint, not from a counsellor's. But how else can they be expected to make judgements if the counsellor has not explained his viewpoint? Those who are willing to give the counsellor a trial run before pronouncing judgement will also be disappointed unless the counsellor has taken great care to gain their sympathy for and their understanding of his work and methods.

Thus the sorts of questions teachers ask publicly, privately and inwardly when faced with a counsellor for the first time are often based on a series of false expectations which *ipso facto* are bound to lead to dissatisfaction with the counsellor. The new counsellor may be caricatured mentally as an almighty power or as a ridiculous mouse. It is natural for staff to have mixed feelings about the counsellor at first but if this state of fantasy and disillusion continues, it simply means that the counsellor is not doing the job properly.

In the present stage of the development of counselling, the onus of proof as to what a counsellor is still rests with the counsellors. Everybody has been to school and everybody knows (or thinks he knows) what a teacher's job is. Nobody knows exactly what a counsellor's job is and it is up to the counsellor to demonstrate this constantly.

A counsellor who assumes that others understand his work is making a false assumption. He must tell the staff what he is trying to do and why; to adapt the old teaching adage, 'He must tell them, he must tell them again and he must tell them he's told them.' What is more, the counsellor must be seen to be what he claims to be; ultimately the service will be used or misused according to its quality. In the meantime while the service is being established it is important for the counsellor himself to disclaim any impression or illusion that he is either superhuman or omnipotent, for he certainly is neither. He is just one member of a team of people, each with a complementary and supplementary role. The counsellor who has given the impression that *he* will solve the children's problems is asking to be discredited; the teacher who has sent a child to the counsellor because he is difficult and finds that after several weeks' counselling the child is not better but more difficult than ever is liable to be very annoyed with the counsellor. It is important therefore for staff to realize for example that it is not uncommon for a pupil's behaviour to deteriorate after counselling has begun, partly because the pupil may be releasing and trying to come to terms with feelings he finds uncomfortable to face. It is important also for staff to accept that there is no guarantee of success unless the pupil himself wants to improve. Counselling does not obviate the necessity for ordinary classroom discipline, which should continue as usual.

A counsellor who has not educated the staff about his role and methods is at fault. To establish the teacher/counsellor relationship takes as much care and time, if not more, as establishing a viable pupil/counsellor relationship. Even if the counsellor is under no illusions about what he can achieve, it may happen that despite his protestations and definitions, certain staff will persist in regarding him as someone who will 'cure' problems. The answer here is for the teacher and counsellor to talk over a problem together and work out in discussion their respective roles. This stops the teacher from devaluing his own importance. It helps him to see the counsellor in perspective–as someone who can be useful but who has decidedly limited value and virtually no powers as all.

In order to maintain good relationships with the staff it is important for a counsellor to point out at all times the difference if any between their expectations and his practice. For example staff, like the children, may try to manipulate the counsellor: 'This girl wants to leave and she should not. Could you sort her out?' 'This girl has a very close relationship with her boyfriend. Could you find out what they are up to?' When the counsellor neither persuades the girl to stay on at school nor reports on her sexual behaviour, resentment may well set in unless the counsellor has already explained that his role is neither to persuade children to take certain courses of action nor to spy on their private lives.

Having a counsellor on the staff does not prevent teachers using for themselves the techniques of persuasion and direct questioning. But a counsellor who is really the arm of the law in subtle disguise is doing his clients a grave disservice. His first duty is to serve the needs of his clients; he must therefore resist the pressures of his environment to use his service as another, albeit subtle, way of enforcing conformity. The counsellor may hope that after counselling, a child will, as part of his growing maturity, come to accept the responsibilities of the society in which he lives. But there is no built-in guarantee.

If we turn now to what actually happened in our experiment, it will become clear straightaway that the only reason I am able now to issue *caveats* with a certain degree of certainty is that they are born of experience. Our path was by no means as clear then as it seems in retrospect.

The teacher/counsellor relationship in our school went through a series of phases, rather like many a marriage: first the honeymoon, then a short period of semi-illusionment when harsh reality begins to temper over-idealism, then finally a realistic working relationship in which the strengths and weaknesses of both partners are perceived, accepted and blended as harmoniously and constructively as possible.

The counsellor's arrival was hailed with great enthusiasm and a feeling that at last something would be done directly and early with girls who had problems. The counsellor herself shared this euphoric and optimistic mood. The head and the senior staff gave her the warmest of welcomes and did a lot of groundwork in advance. Before the counsellor arrived the head had discussed the idea and the scheme with the staff, individually and collectively; the counsellor had individual discussions with key members of staff, and with all the third year form tutors with whom she was going to deal in particular. The work began enthusiastically. By the end of the first term an important difference of approach between the teaching staff and the counsellor was apparent. The staff wanted to know what could be done to help a particular individual. The counsellor could only say there was nothing to be *done*; everything that could be done had already been done (such as providing free dinners, arranging a school journey etc). What the girl needed was warm but firm relationships with the adults in her life, tasks to do which she could achieve, praise and encouragement for her achievements which might reinforce her positive feelings about herself, avoidance (if possible) of situations in which her negative qualities would be stressed—yet on the other hand no 'extra soft' treatment. In other words the counsellor's approach was less practical and tangible than the teachers' and almost entirely to do with the quality of the relationships between the individual and the people in her life.

The way the teachers handle their relationships with their pupils is something so bound up with their own attitudes and attributes that it is something the counsellor cannot *tell* them to change, any more than she can tell the children to change. This approach is both tactless and ineffectual. It would in any case assume that the counsellor knew the answers and herself had 'superior' attitudes—neither of which is true.

The reaction of the staff to the realization that the counsellor is herself as human and limited as anyone else is a kind of double-take; annoyance that this person doesn't have a simple answer to a complicated question, and that after all the buck still rests with them; then a dawning of positive feelings. If the counsellor does not know the answer then the teacher is still herself the most important person *vis-à-vis* the child; it is the teacher who spends most of her time with the pupil and the counsellor is very much a fringe benefit. The overall responsibility for the child therefore still rests with the teacher; thus the counsellor does not undermine the teacher/pupil relationship. A parallel may be drawn with the counsellor/client relationship. If the counsellor takes over the responsibility of the child or of the teacher, she is not helping them to be more responsible or to take responsibility for themselves, yet in both spheres this is one of her objectives.

The teacher who faces the full extent of her responsibility for a child may in fact increase her own respect for herself as an effective form teacher; through believing in herself in this role, she may *be* a more effective form teacher. The counsellor's role is not to tell her what to do, but exactly as with the clients to get her to talk about what she thinks she might do, to air her feelings, her doubts, her attitudes, her reasons. With teachers as with clients, the counsellor does not know the answer, and it would not really help if she did. The teachers work out their own answers but with the additional sense of perspective, clarity or insight brought about by having voiced their thoughts. The counsellor is not the only person who can provide this non-rebounding sounding board within a school. But again, as with clients, the non-authoritarian, non-judgemental role of the counsellor is occasionally helpful. If you tell your boss you are making a mess of things you may think rightly or wrongly that she will not be able to give you a very good reference; if you can trust the counsellor not to reveal what she is told then there are no repercussions for one's status or future prospects.

At the beginning of the second year of our experiment the counsellors were aware of some hostile undercurrents; it seemed important to face up to these feelings. We arranged a meeting with the third year tutors, during which a great deal of hostility was expressed towards the child guidance clinic, hostility which was in fact really about the counselling service. There was a feeling that nothing changed, nobody improved after treatment, 'they' didn't tell you how to handle a child, 'they' wouldn't tell you anything because everything was confidential, so how could you help?

We realized that in our desire to establish a confidential client-centred service, we had at this stage neglected our relationships with the staff. We had been on good terms with the staff but we had not worked out our relationship with them sufficiently and we had not communicated with them well enough, so afraid were we of damaging our relationship with the pupils. This explosive meeting cleared the air for everybody. Through the discussion the staff began to see more clearly what the counsellors were trying to do. From that moment the staff and the counsellors began to perceive each other more realistically. By the end of the second year of the experiment, the staff began to use the counsellors extremely well, and the counsellors began to use the resources of the staff as a whole more effectively in the service of their clients. Realism had set in.

As a result of the group discussion the counsellors realized that it was not good enough to assume good relationships and good communication with the staff. Good communication needs proper channels of communication and the only way to ensure proper channels of communication is with official structure and timetabling. A chance meeting over lunch or in the staffroom is not the moment to begin serious discussion of an individual. For a start nothing so important should be left to chance or it might never happen. Second a hasty public interchange provides neither the calm nor the privacy essential for a well considered discussion of a child's needs. A rash, off the cuff comment about a child by a counsellor or by a teacher may well give an incomplete or false impression which is damaging to the child, particularly if the comment is also overheard by a member of staff sitting nearby who is even less acquainted with the whole truth.

It was for these reasons that we began to structure most carefully the staff/counsellor contacts. Naturally there is informal contact at break, over lunch and between lessons, but if there is something serious and lengthy to discuss, then the counsellor may use the social occasion to make an appointment for a proper discussion, rather than embark on something complicated in a few hasty moments. Sometimes the counsellor arranges to see a certain member of staff at break. The advantage of working in this way is that teacher and counsellor are able to give thought to the discussion in advance. In particular the counsellor has decided professionally, not on the spur of the moment, how much she is able to say about a child, and what the purpose of the discussion is.

It would be wrong to give the impression here that the counsellors never talk to the staff except by arrangement. It is essential for the counsellor to seize every opportunity for communicating with teaching colleagues, to miss no opportunity for saying, 'And how is Naomi?' Teachers will sometimes spontaneously proffer the information that a client or former client is going through a bad patch; prompting by the counsellor forms an extra safety net. More important than the interchange of information is the maintenance of a warm, trusting relationship between the teacher and counsellor, and a feeling that both are working together for the good of the child.

As a result of setting up proper channels of teacher/counsellor communication, staff attitudes to counselling became more realistic. This is partly a function of time. Whatever system is adopted, the efficacy of a counselling service will not be accepted by the staff overnight. We found that it took the best part of two years for the service to be realistically perceived, emotionally accepted and wisely used. Apart from the few members of staff who have always been sceptical of the service and steered clear of the counsellors, the staff/counsellor relationship has continued to grow in strength and understanding. It is not only that the staff understand what the counsellors are trying to do, but that the counsellors too are beginning to have a clearer idea of their function.

The organization of staff/counsellor relationships in the school

Thus alongside the system of group discussions organized for third year girls there is a careful scheme of staff contact. At the beginning of each academic year the head introduces the counsellors to the staff as a whole and explains their role. The mistress in charge of the third year calls a meeting of all third year tutors after school at which the counsellors again explain the pattern of the group work, their role and way of working. Any questions are answered or discussed. This again is not enough: approximately half a term is spent with each form and so form tutors whose forms are to be seen at the end of the academic year will have forgotten what it is all about by then. It is also more conducive to a good teacher/counsellor relationship for the counsellor to see the tutor individually again before starting work with her form. So the counsellor makes contact with the form tutor just before the group discussions with her form begin to remind her again of the scheme; to explain how to get the girls to divide into groups and why; to discuss which lessons it is most practical for the girls to miss in order to come for discussions; to ask the form tutor to negotiate and excuse these alterations in timetable for the next three weeks; to discuss in general terms what this particular form is like. Sometimes the form tutor will tell the counsellor which girls to look out for. But this is not always helpful to the counselling relationship as it can have the effect of inhibiting or prejudicing the counsellor. On the whole it is preferable to take the group without prior knowledge.

After the three weeks of discussion groups and the preliminary interview the counsellor spends one or two periods discussing the form with the year mistress and form tutor. This is something which was not done in the beginning except rather casually. The year mistress and the form tutor are the people most intimately concerned with the day-to-day life of the individual pupil. They have a good impression of what a girl is like and whether she shows any signs of strain and they can provide the counsellor with useful reality based information which helps the counsellor in assessing whether there is a need for a referral. By seeing both key pastoral carers at once the counsellor ensures that the level of communication with each is the same. This avoids the situation of one member of the trio saying—or feeling—'But you didn't tell me about that particular difficulty. If I'd known, I could have done more.' The year mistress and the form tutor contribute their impressions freely to the discussion, the counsellor only says what does not break confidentiality, though she may well have a child's permission to pass on information on a confidential basis if this really seems appropriate and helpful.

More often than not the year mistress and form tutor know a lot more than the counsellor about the child's background. If they come out with the facts that Betty's parents are separated, that there are six children, that Betty is always late for school and looks tired and undernourished, then there is little point in the counsellor keeping this information, which the girl has also explained in confidence, as if it were a deadly secret. It may be something which the staff responsible for the child already know, but which is *not* common knowledge. The form tutor usually knows whether a girl is coping with her life or finding it a strain, though she may not always know why. Sometimes a girl who the form teacher knows needs extra help may write a very non-committal note, and not come forward for counselling. In this case counselling is not thrust upon her, though the form tutor may decide to make a more determined and direct approach herself to get to the root of her troubles. Because a girl does not choose to come for counselling does not mean that no one can help her. She may prefer to talk to someone else, or she may already be under the wing of a social worker.

The triangular discussions are held in the counsellor's room, not in the staffroom: this is to ensure greater privacy and a relaxed atmosphere. Every member of each form is discussed though in most cases there is little to say. In order to establish what is already known about each girl the counsellor asks the staff to talk first. The counsellor has already checked with the girl concerned whether the school knows about separated parents or a handicapped brother or whatever it is; thus the counsellor knows whether it is important to the girl that this family secret be kept secret. Occasionally parents have confided in the form tutor without the girl's knowledge and so the tutor tells the counsellor what the counsellor would otherwise have kept secret. It may be important to the girl's own pride and self-esteem to feel her home life and school life are kept separate, even if in fact they are not. In this rather delicate situation, the counsellor has to remember that betraying confidences is not just a question of relating facts: if she is lulled into a sense of false security by thinking that the staff already know about this particular child and that there is little point therefore in being discreet, she has to remember not to reveal attitudes or opinions which may be more a betrayal than the hard facts.

The discussion between the year mistress, form tutor and counsellor takes place after the group discussions have ended and all the girls have had their brief routine interview. This is a good time for the contact, because the counsellor has not yet begun counselling proper. It is natural for staff to want to know *why* a child wants to come for counselling, particularly if it is someone rather unexpected. At this stage all the counsellor knows is that Jenny wants to come for counselling but she does not really know why. It is therefore easier for the counsellor to withstand the pressures of the staff's natural curiosity. If later on it is appropriate for the tutor to know why Jenny is being counselled the counsellor will tell her why with the child's permission. Without doubt it is the counsellor's duty, in the interests of the child, to *communicate* with the form teacher; bad communication might set up hostility, resentment or jealousy in the tutor, which in turn could adversely affect the child. But communicating does not mean telling all; the staff are not led to expect an explanation of why a girl is coming for counselling, and if they receive an explanation it is because it is something that they know already or that the child does not mind their knowing.

After the discussion of each form the counsellor will keep in touch with the form tutor. The counsellor depends on the tutor to let her know of any particular developments in the work or behaviour of her clients or former clients. The discussion of a child can help both teacher and counsellor to develop their insight about her. The form tutor also helps the counsellor by handing out appointment slips to the girls and excusing them from lessons when they come for individual counselling.

The appointment slips are written out and distributed by the deputy head. This is logical as she has particular responsibility for the third and fourth years with whom the counsellors mostly work;

she also has particular responsibility for the timetable. Thus in one action she keeps track of both the counsellors and the counselled. She has an opportunity to check on the way the counsellor is spending her time; she is also able to check that a girl does not repeatedly miss the same lesson. The counsellor will in fact write out a suggested timetable and list of appointments which is usually accepted.

The official blessing given to the appointment by this arrangement helps the staff to accept that this is a genuine excuse which is therefore not to be questioned. The appointment slip, which the girl takes with her to the lesson she must miss, also acts as an official pass for getting out of the lesson. This avoids any suspicion that 'going to see Mrs Jones' is a euphemism for having a smoke or roaming the corridors. If a spontaneous interview has to be arranged the counsellor herself will write a note to excuse the girl from her lesson. When a girl asks to leave a lesson the staff do not ask the girl why, though they may well ask themselves this question. Any complaints about lessons being missed go through the form tutor to the deputy head if necessary. These are not very frequent; when they do occur they are usually for good reasons and the timetable is adjusted accordingly. The departure of a girl for an official counselling session is intended to be treated as unobtrusively as possible. As far as it is possible to ascertain by questioning staff and pupils individual counselling is normally accepted without annoyance from the staff or gossip from the girls. The longer the service has been established and proved, the more this is likely to be the case.

Counselling and school records

It is pertinent to ask at this stage what contribution the counsellors make to the school records and what happens to all the valuable information they collect about the girls. In many counselling schemes, the counsellor himself takes responsibility for setting up and maintaining the school record cards; he collects and collates information from the primary school, interviews all pupils in the first year and adds his own comments plus any information about pupils' backgrounds to the card. This can be a very useful function, but it is not a function which is compatible with the particular kind of counselling service we have established in our school. The existing system of official record-keeping is that the primary school profile, the interview notes, and any correspondence between home and school are kept in filing cabinets along with a new record card of each girl's academic and social progress which is maintained by form tutors. Form tutors have access to the records of their form; any particularly confidential matters are restricted to the medical records which are kept locked in the medical room and are not accessible to tutors without special permission.

The counsellor's records are kept separate from the other records and are regarded as completely confidential. The autobiographical notes were written by the girls on this understanding; they are never on any account shown to members of staff however innocuous they may be. The counsellor's own case notes are equally confidential, their purpose being to help the counsellor remember and understand the details of her client's case. The counsellors have a filing cabinet which locks, and to which no other member of staff has access; this includes the head who accepts, in a way not all heads would accept, that she does not have to know everything about each and every child. It is important to add here that the head and deputy head know a great deal about many girls which they too keep confidential. Unless the girl concerned however happens to be on the counsellor's books there is little point in their passing on information. If the counsellor is already seeing a girl it seems unlikely that she would not be told about the matter directly by the girl. Confidentiality works both ways. Discretion is by no means the prerogative of the counsellor.

The counsellors rarely add anything to the official records of the school because they are extremely cautious about the possible effects of labelling children as problems. If children are generally difficult the school is already well aware of this; if they are generally well adjusted there is no need to cast doubts on this by alluding to their problems. In a case where action, such as referral to a specialist agency, is taken, then this is usually known to the school and noted accordingly. In cases where the problem can be sorted out between the client and the counsellor and is entirely private and personal (that is, in no way affecting the girl's school life) no note at all is made in the school records. Form tutors know of course which of their girls come to see the counsellor. Tutors are asked to let the counsellor know if the girls become involved with any other agency. The counsellor then advises whether it is in the girl's interest for her to contact the agency with the child's permission. This kind of co-operation is particularly important with the careers officer and the school doctor. The counsellors, guided by the form tutors, try not to miss an opportunity for constructive communication where it is in the girl's interest and with the girl's blessing.

Teachers do not always accept readily the idea of confidential counsellor records. There is a strong view within the teaching profession that the counsellor is doing a grave disservice by sitting on all the valuable information she has gathered. Teachers argue, with good reason, that they cannot help a child if they do not know what is the matter; that if they understood a child's problems, they could deal with them more sympathetically. But in the first place the counsellor is not in any way coming between or taking over the normal means of communication between teacher and pupil: it is still an important part of each form tutor's duty to get to know her pupils as well as possible. In the second place a child with problems is not necessarily helped by being treated any differently from other children, either more leniently or more punitively. Fair and equal treatment for all would surely be one of the first demands of any pupil power movement.

The conflicts provoked among teachers by the concept of confidentiality are usually out of proportion. Form tutors are usually well informed about their pupils' backgrounds, which reduces the amount of truly confidential information to a small proportion. There is never any point in burdening the staff with information which has no bearing at all on the way the child is behaving in school; when it is relevant to school behaviour it is very rare (never, in my experience) for the counsellor not to get the child's permission to explain the situation; or better still to get the child to say something herself.

Confidentiality does not equal non-communication. It is possible to communicate to staff that a child is having a difficult time at home without going into details, though there *is* a danger that hinting darkly at problems might set a form tutor's imagination boggling into fantasies more horrific than reality. It is best to get the child's permission for a straightforward honest statement. The communication of irrelevant knowledge can be both useless and damaging to the individual; the communication of confidential knowledge to staff merely provides them with a blunt weapon. If they are told they must not use this knowledge they are then left with a feeling of frustration and impotence; if they are tempted to use or unwittingly use what they are told in confidence there is a betrayal of the individual. If the matter really is confidential it is confidential; a compromise of half truth helps neither the pupil nor the staff.

If we take any educational issue it is clear that there are advantages and disadvantages in every scheme. If we think of streaming versus non-streaming or house groups versus year groups for example we must admit that there are good arguments for and against each side.

Our confidential self-referral service has certain advantages: our clients want to be helped and they trust us. When they talk freely it is precisely because they are confident of our trustworthiness. If they are not confident of our integrity they will not talk. If they do not mind the staff knowing they will talk to them; they may talk to a counsellor as well because she has more time.

One of the disadvantages of our scheme is in the very few cases when a girl actually says, 'I can tell you this because you have said you won't tell anyone, and you mustn't–otherwise I won't tell you.' At some stage, preferably at the beginning, the counsellor has to make it clear that because of the child's age and the counsellor's responsibility to the child, to her family, to the school and to society, there *is* a limit to the amount of explosive material the counsellor can accept and sit on passively. On the other hand if the counsellor has the strength not to take precipitate action she may find that the client will change her mind later and ask for something to be done. The prohibition was more to test out the counsellor than to prevent action.

If for any reason the client does lose confidence in the counsellor, then there is no hope of further counselling until confidence has been restored. With staff-referrals the counsellor/client relationship is generally more tenuous at first, for the pupil may imagine that the staff are trying to manipulate her through the counsellor. When staff and counsellor are both involved in helping a particular child it is important not to confuse their different roles. The staff may need to take punitive action or to send for a parent because of a girl's bad behaviour. If the girl becomes confused and thinks this has come about because she has talked to the counsellor, then the counselling relationship is lost. Plain dealing rather than double dealing usually clears up this kind of confusion, though a girl who is ambivalent about getting help may well seize on any opportunity to avoid facing her own problems.

Although our service is basically designed to encourage self-referrals, staff-referrals are often made. We find that referrals made in the first and second years are not always as effective as referrals of older girls. This is partly because the girls are young and less able to take responsibility for themselves in the way we would like; partly because they are not quite sure who or what the counsellor is, although this has been explained to them by staff and counsellors. Any girl who has been through the third year groups has a good idea of the way the counsellor works. For example Sandra was referred by the staff in the fourth year for 'playing truant, being disobedient and generally getting into trouble'. Had she not been a member of a group the previous year when she had, in fact, been calm and relatively trouble-free, it is highly likely that she would have sat sullen and uncommunicative before yet another adult who looked as if she was going to 'deal' with her. She knew the counsellor already and knew the terms of reference under which the counsellor worked and she was able to communicate very quickly the kind of strain she was feeling in her relationship with her family. This is something she had not made clear in the disciplinary setting. She needed to go to the child guidance clinic; the interview with the counsellor confirmed what the school already suspected—that there was more to this than adolescent high spirits. A referral to the clinic was made forthwith, the girl herself accepting the need for this kind of help.

This example shows that the counsellor can miss many opportunities for helping girls unless she is backed up by the staff. The staff can help enormously by reminding girls who are having difficulties about the counselling service: if the girl then accepts that counselling might be useful, progress can be made. If the girl does not like the idea of counselling or the counsellor, then some other solution, as in the days *before* counsellors existed, has to be tried. Counselling is only one of many possible solutions to any problem, and may not always be appropriate. It is an extra source of help, but it is by no means a cure-all.

Criticism of staff and school organization

What does a counsellor do if a group or an individual begins to criticize the school regime or individual members of staff? This may be what the girls themselves want to know, which is why they are trying it on. The counsellor's way of dealing with it will be astutely judged by the girls. The counsellor who is so insecure as to sacrifice her own integrity and professional standards in order to be popular and 'in' with the girls is not only disloyal to her teaching colleagues she is also soon seen through by the pupils who will not respect her for her lack of standards. In this situation the objectivity of the counsellor and her role as an outsider are of paramount importance. Her way of dealing with the situation is simple and firm: she does not become involved; she does not take sides but remains outside; she may ask a few questions designed to provoke a consideration of the feelings of the staff or the reasoning behind the ruling but she puts the responsibility for action firmly back with the individuals concerned. On no account does she take upon herself the role of trade union negotiator. If the grievance is genuine, the children's own appointed leader can take the matter up with the authorities concerned or raise the issue in school council. It is amazing how many grievances disappear spontaneously at this point. When it becomes known on the third year bush telegraph that there is no joy in trying to get the counsellor to support the children against the staff, then baiting the counsellor loses its appeal. Most children understand and accept readily the way the school is run and why. Those who do feel unjustly treated may on reflection be able to see how their own behaviour and attitudes have contributed to this. Raising this kind of issue with the counsellor is therefore an uncomfortable process for it brings the individual up against her own limitations and does not allow the school to remain a convenient scapegoat.

Personal criticisms of members of staff usually reflect the emotional needs of the pupils more than the attributes of the teacher herself. This becomes clear when the same member of staff is praised by one pupil and criticized by another, perhaps even for the same quality, such as being strict. Occasionally a teacher may be the victim of antagonism really intended for an unsatisfactory mother. The pupil/teacher relationship in such a case can be the source of great strain and conflict, not only for the individuals concerned but for the whole class. This tension can be relieved if the child is able to ventilate her strong feelings. The counsellor recognizes these feelings for what they are: not the true situation necessarily but an expression of the child's emotional needs. If the cause for concern really lay within the teacher, then the majority of the form would feel this way. Once the child has expressed her anger she may begin to get the situation into perspective. If the child tries to manipulate the counsellor to side against the teacher she will soon stop when she finds it gets her nowhere.

The teacher who is being used as an emotional scapegoat by a pupil must find this a great worry and even begin to lose confidence. It can therefore be reassuring to the teacher if she has the courage to face the counsellor with her side of the problem, to realize that this is not simply a case of bad handling on her part but something much more complex. The counsellor can help restore the teacher's self-confidence and sense of perspective as well as the pupil's; the counsellor does this in the same way as she helps the pupil—that is, not by prescribing the answer but by listening to what she says, accepting and respecting her as a person with professional skills. The teacher who has a difficult child to deal with may be afraid to reveal the extent of her difficulties in case it makes her appear inadequate. The counsellor can make a helpful comment to open the way to communication. By facing the issue the teacher may be able to assess more realistically the way the pupil is playing on an emotional weak point of hers and gain the strength to deal more resiliently as well as more sympathetically with this particular pupil.

What does the counsellor do if several pupils criticize a member of staff independently of each other and when there does appear to be some justification in the accusations? Does the counsellor report this to the head? She certainly does not. This sort of breach of confidence would be completely unprofessional; it would also be unnecessary. Any counsellor who imagines that the head and her senior colleagues are not aware of the strengths and weaknesses of members of staff is suffering from delusions of grandeur. It is part of the head's job to know her staff, to develop and inspire the best in them. The counsellor is not going to improve staff performance any more than children's by reporting them to the authorities. This kind of judgemental role can only undermine the teacher/counsellor relationship. The counsellor must not use what the children have said about a teacher, partly because it may be a distortion of the truth, partly because this does nothing to improve teacher/pupil relationships. If the member of staff concerned comes to the counsellor to talk about her difficulties this must be kept as confidential as any interview with a girl.

It is only when a teacher brings forward to the counsellor some of the problems she is facing in the classroom that the counsellor has any role to play in improving staff performance. But the counsellor's role in the staffroom is not to be overlooked. The counsellor who has learnt to work discreetly and unobtrusively with staff may do much, indirectly, to help the staff develop their own strengths and minimize their own weaknesses. By keeping in touch with the staff the counsellor also ensures that she herself does not forget the difficulties of the classroom situation; she does not know the answers any more than they do but these can be worked out in discussion.

Staff/group discussions

Sometimes a particular girl is causing trouble with everybody who teaches her. This may be a girl who is not particularly amenable to counselling. In this sort of situation we have found it invaluable to get together all the members of staff who teach the girl. In one notable case a second year girl, Barbara, was causing great concern. She was very sensitive to any mild rebuke and would respond to any direction by any teacher with a great show of aggression and fuss. Every member of staff was suffering at her hands, except for the drama and housecraft teachers in whose lessons there was a greater degree of freedom and self-expression. The staff meeting was held after school, over cups of tea. The counsellor said that it was difficult to get at the root of this particular girl's problems, and that it might help in understanding Barbara if everybody would say something about her. One by one staff listed misdeeds, annoyances, rudeness, belligerence. The counsellor began to regret having convened the meeting, fearing that the discussion was simply inflaming bad feelings against Barbara. Then suddenly there came a great wave of sympathy for Barbara; one after the other the staff expressed concern for how Barbara must feel in this position of being constantly criticized and devalued. The counsellor said that it was best to wait and see how Barbara developed from then on; if nothing changed there would have to be a referral to the child guidance clinic.

The extraordinary thing is that from that moment Barbara began to improve. Why was this? She grew up a little and this helped; she was also greatly helped by the staff as a whole, who mustered just that little extra tolerance needed to carry her over this passing phase. There is nothing so depressing and so reinforcing of one's sense of worthlessness as being constantly criticized. The staff tried, not to be lenient with her, but to look for the good in her and avoid collisions between their authority and her need to assert her own. In this case it had proved impossible to work with Barbara's attitudes to her social environment; it proved worthwhile working with the attitudes of the school to Barbara. These are not necessarily mutually exclusive processes; in some cases it is worth trying both. It is worth noting that in neither approach is the counsellor altering Barbara's *actual* environment—the counsellor is not a juggler of externals.

The counsellor's role in school policy

Although in our scheme we have taken great care to keep the counsellor outside the main stream of school organization and discipline we have realized that to insulate the counsellor totally from school policy does not help her to help her clients. She must not identify with the school powers, but she must not be so isolated from them as to become alienated. If she is to assess what is normal behaviour in a client, she must know what is normally expected of her and why. The counsellor who herself does not know or understand what school policy is may quite unwittingly make a comment which goes against the objectives of the school. It makes it harder for her to retain the neutrality and objectivity she claims, if she only hears the children's remarks about what is going on. The counsellor has to keep her feet on the ground, even if she does not use them very much. Whether or not the counsellor agrees with everything the school is doing she has, like all the staff, a duty not to undermine what the school is trying to achieve. The easiest way for her to understand this is for her to attend and participate in staff meetings or discussions. It may even be helpful to the staff for her opinion to be sought on some new organizational scheme: the counsellor's role as outside observer of the school's social structure gives her an opportunity for an objective assessment of the effects of policy on social behaviour. The counsellor may be wrong, but it is both healthier and more constructive for her to put forward her view for consideration alongside the views of the rest of the staff.

The counsellor then has a useful viewpoint to contribute on decisions of policy and should therefore participate in staff discussions. On the other hand, general staff meetings are not the moment for the counsellor to add to the general discussion of an individual child. This risks misrepresentation, distortion and breach of confidentiality. A properly convened discussion is a different matter. If the counsellor does contribute to discussions on school policy the only danger for her clients is that she will begin to identify too closely with the school system and start to succumb to pressures to make children conform. If the counsellor is aware of this possible side effect, she is more likely to retain her objectivity and sense of perspective.

Conclusion

It is entirely natural for teachers to feel ambivalent about counselling at first. The counsellor too will feel insecure and needs the full support of the head and staff in setting up a counselling scheme. Consultation at all times is essential to ensure good communication and good relationships.

However the goodwill and support of the staff are not enough to ensure a constructive working relationship between staff and counsellor. The counsellor has to take the initiative in defining and explaining at every opportunity her role and function. There needs to be regular discussion, properly convened, between appropriate members of staff and the counsellor, to ensure the maximum co-operation, understanding and efficiency. Co-operation with the staff at every level does not go against the counsellor's role as a trustworthy outsider, provided the counsellor is sufficiently disciplined professionally to remain objective. Through working out together their complementary roles, the teacher and counsellor are both able to help the individual child more. Discussing his own difficulties with a counsellor sometimes helps a teacher to improve his own self-insight and techniques of pastoral care. Members of staff who have natural counselling skills can continue to deploy them, with the added self-assurance and effectiveness gained from their discussion with the counsellor. This relieves the counsellor of the burden of dealing with cases which can be perfectly well handled by form tutors; it enhances the role of the form tutor; it spreads the effects of the counsellor's specialized training skills and philosophy throughout the staff, thus ensuring an even greater unity of purpose between teacher and counsellor and leaving the counsellor more time to deal with those cases in which his specialized training and his role as outsider are important to and needed by the client. Thus the counsellor's work with the staff is almost as important as the work with the children in furthering his general objectives. A relationship between staff and counsellor built on mutual respect, confidence, trust and reciprocal co-operation is essential to an effective counselling service. A counsellor who neglects relationships with the staff is doing his clients a grave disservice.

Chapter 6

The adolescent world

How do adolescents see the rest of us? How do they feel about the way we behave, the way we handle them? What are their hopes and fears, their needs and their problems, real and imagined? Having explained the mechanics of our counselling service, and the ways in which we established a working relationship with the girls and with the staff, I want now to discuss the girls' feelings and problems. This will lead in turn to illustration of the ways we work with staff, parents, and the social welfare agencies. There is a great deal of overlap between the problems expressed in the groups and the problems expressed by individuals; thus the sorts of comments made in groups and in the autobiographical notes can form a useful background to individual problems; they can also give non-adolescents greater insight into the adolescent's feelings. They provide a glimpse of the various ways adolescents currently view the adult world. It is not easy for adults to keep in touch with the 'teen scene' at a realistic level. Some adults are rather intimidated by the modern adolescent, some are jealous, some bewildered, some belligerent, some reactionary, others are permissive to the point of appearing not to care what happens. It is hoped that the comments made by the girls in their autobiographical notes will illustrate the kinds of feelings and problems experienced by normal adolescent girls who do not need counselling. Most of the comments speak for themselves, though they would repay close scrutiny and detailed discussion. In quoting these notes I have been careful to remove any details which would make them identifiable. The spelling and phrasing are given as in the originals. I think they give a vivid and valid view of the way girls of 13-14 feel. James Hemming's book *Problems of Adolescent Girls*, based largely on letters girls wrote to magazines, has a similar flavour and reveals a similar range of problems.[1]

Parents

My mother is a very nice, kind person and she'll do almost anything for me and I've never hid anything from her, and don't think I ever will, no matter what.

I have to be in by eight o'clock every single night. My Dad's very strict—I wanted to go to a party but my dad wouldn't let me. My mum won't let me do anything and I get sick and tired of it but I know its for my own good but she treats me like a five year old. My mum worries about me with boys in case anything happens, and I could hate her sometimes but I feel sorry for my dad.

I don't think they like me as much as my sisters because I get blamed for everything.

I find that I get fed-up with my parents when they start to row and this usually leaves me with no place to go to get out of the house.

When it comes to getting up in the mornings, both my parents start calling me and shouting at me. My dad bellows at me as if he were still in the RAF.

One thing I hate about my mum, say if there's boys standing outside the verandah or in the streets, she starts up a fight with me and sought of chucks me out and tries to show me up in front of them. I've got that feeling that she don't seem to want me to grow up, like not going out with boys, she sought of seems to think I go out of my way to go out with them, but I have not been out with a boy yet.

My mum is very strict and sometimes I go to bed at 8 o'clock and read to get away from her. If I go out before tea, I have to be back by 6 o'clock and I'm not aloud out any more.

I am staying on at school. It was my own decision. As my mum said, only I know what I want to do.

My mother can be very nagging if she wants to. I can't stand this and it usually ends with me walking out of the room.

I am allowed out whenever I want to which is not very often as there is not any clubs or dances where I live and you usually have to travel to get anywhere interesting.

My life is quite unhappy as my parents keep on at me.

I smoke and my mum knows, because what is the use of doing it behind their backs so you might as well do it in front of them.

My dad is very nice to me sometimes but suddenly changes and goes all moody. I'm not yet allowed to go out with boys but I always do and we always have rows over this.

My parents are rather old and getting rather moany—my mother is nearly always moany especially in the morning. My father I hardly ever see. I get on alright with my father because he is always nice to me and hardly ever grumbles. My mother though, always says don't do this, don't do that and so I always feel as though I'm in the wrong.

My mother is strange in a way, one minute she is helpful and will say things like 'never you mind, you're growing up' and the next minute she will go off in a flying temper because I am growing up. I know this is because she is starting the change, but it doesn't help and I never know what mood she will be in. Every now and then she gets into a temper because I never go out. I would like to, but somehow I just can't mix and make friends.

My mother and father don't trust me at night.

My mum goes to work and so we all have to muck in with the jobs: this is usually when the fights occur.

My dad goes mad when I stop out with boys. I am not allowed to go anywhere unless there is a reason.

My mother don't mind me going out with boys but she hits me when I come in late.

My father's not bad, but he's only interested in my education and my mother don't like me going around with boys. I have three boy friends.

My mother worries a lot and she is always fussing.

My mother wants me to have every opportunity possible where education is concerned as she did not have such opportunities when she was at school. I find we don't understand each other very well.

I never lie to my father as I think this only makes one untrustworthy and he respects me for this.

My parents quite often get on my nerves when they don't understand our modern ways.

I look after myself really and I'm just in the house at night. When I am old enough I want to leave home.

I find it hard to please both my parents at once.

My mother works part-time. My father disagrees with her work as he thinks she should be at home in case of emergency.

I don't know if its my imagination or not but I think my parents honestly don't understand children.

I am the only child. My parents and I discuss things and we do not have any real secrets from each other. If I ask them anything they answer it whatever it may be. I find it very easy to talk to my parents especially my mother. They are very understanding and fair. I don't think they spoil me, and if there is something I do not want to do and they want me to do, they say, that I must do it and if I don't they get annoyed.

Comment

Although negative comments about parents were the exception rather than the rule, nevertheless it seems that it is not easy for parents to deal with their teenage daughters or vice versa. Many of the complaints made by the girls were clearly reality based and not just symptoms of adolescent rebellion. Over-possessiveness, jealousy, moodiness, bad temper, rivalry, constant nagging, anxiety, lack of affection or communication, favouritism of other siblings, apparent indifference—these are the sorts of characteristics which make for problem parents. It is important to note that most children did not criticize their parents: usually there was no comment, occasionally a positive comment. Nevertheless these examples, though highly coloured, are typical of the way many girls of 13-14 years of age see their parents. The group discussions confirmed this.

Siblings

My three sisters are married so there is just me and my brother. He's always bossing me around and telling me off.

I have one brother who is seventeen years old and we do not get along very well, we are always arguing and fighting but he always wins the fighting for he is much stronger.

My little brother is a mongolian child. This upsets me when people joke about it.

I have one sister but long for an older brother but naturally this was not possible as I was the first child born.

My brother's at work. He's alright, but he gets a bit moody, still probably its because he hasn't really got a girl-friend.

My elder sister of 16 is very handy as she takes the same size as I do and I am nearly always on the borrow.

My sister is 11. She is always causing trouble for me. She will do something and blame it on to me. When my mother goes out she will never do a thing I ask her. Every time she passes me she kicks and hits me. But my parents take no notice of what I say.

My sister is 8 and quite a problem because she asks about babies and where they come from and I wonder if I tell her too much sometimes.

I have one sister who is 20. She is bossy and seems to think that I am lazy, stupid and horrible. She also tries to and does hit me, but seeing as I am growing up to her height, every time she goes to hit me, I warn her off.

My sister is 7 and she often gets on my nerves, so much in fact that I could wring her neck.

I don't get on well with my brother. I am treated as the baby of the family and I rather resent this.

My younger brother is spoilt by my mother, most probably because he is the youngest and she can't fuss my elder brother and me, he usually gets away with a lot of things whereas my brother and I don't.

I hate my brother because he is always showing off when my mates call for me.

I am not as clever as my sister, but I find it very difficult to make my parents, especially my mother, understand.

My sister is a nuisance as she plays her records after me everywhere I go, and she shares a bedroom with me and dirties it up, and also when I decide to go to bed late she stays up too and annoys me. She writes on my books and scribbles on my pictures. She is 8. My big brother is 19. I like him because he tells me whether to get different clothes and whether they suit me, he lets me use his record player, tape recorder and records.

I share my bedroom with my sister and this sometimes causes trouble between her and myself, her being neat and tidy and I not up to her standards.

I've got one brother who is 19, he sometimes gets on my nerves although I become very friendly towards him roundabout Xmas time and my birthday.

Comment

In my experience the girls who wrote the longest pieces about their siblings did not feel the problems as much as it appeared, and having expressed themselves in this dramatic way they had relieved their feelings and did not want to dwell on them longer. Where problems with siblings appear to be serious they are more usually symptoms of problems in relationships with parents. The girls who verbalize their negative feelings so easily are usually equally able to look at the positive side and cheerfully admit for example that they for their part provoke their siblings beyond endurance and deserve all the bad treatment they get. Most of the girls have not got their problems out of proportion and if and when they have elaborated them to interest me, they usually leave it at that. I have not in fact quoted cases which led to sustained supportive work.

Grandparents

My nan won't let me play pop music because she can't stand it.

I live with my nan also. I find her moans are dreadful to hear. I am told I do not do enough for my mother. Sometimes I get so wild I stalk out of the room.

One thing I can't stand is being told I'm talking rubbish just because I'm younger than the person I'm talking to and I don't like people making excuses for old people and saying, 'Well, she's old you know.'

Nan's very nice but she too often reminds me that if it wasn't for her she doesn't know where I would be. This only happens when she's annoyed with me and I don't want to do something for her. Still I expect she's entitled to be like that. Apart from her occasional moans she's very nice and kind and generous.

We all get on, except with Nan. She treats everyone like slaves, dominates all the money and only dishes it out as she sees fit. She gives me lots of money and I suppose she loves me, but I feel that if she would stop making everyone else's life a misery that I might love her in return.

I am the only child and my parents and I live with my father's mother. This is not a bind to us like it would be to some people, but I couldn't imagine living without my grandmother.

My sister and I do not get on very well with my grandad. He is always telling us of what he used to do when he was young, and was always in at 8.30. And now he expects me to be the same. He always wants to know where we are going who we are going with, what time we will be back.

Comment

In fact only one or two girls in each form have grandparents as well as parents to contend with. The girls' comments speak for themselves.

Friends

I go around with one friend. We go out to parties and enjoy ourselves, but she is a blond and very pretty and all the boys look at her, but I find her personality very boring. The boys that do speak to her find out what she is like and then don't think so much of her.

I am very shy, especially when there are boys about. I go all hot and get butterflies in my tummy, but I do like them.

I do not go out with boys although I notice them. I expect I shall start going out with them next year. At the moment I feel I am a little too young.

I have a big problem though, so many boys say they like me, but I don't like them.

I have a boy-friend who is much older than me. My mother does not know about him and I am afraid she will stop me seeing him if she knows. He knows I am only 13.

I like boys, but I am very left out when in a group of girls, and probably thats why I do not go out a lot.

I am very boy-shy. Perhaps this is because there are not many young people of my age where I live. The people are 19-20 or over, or about 6 years old and under.

My interests (if you can call it that) are mostly boys. I get on well with boys, and I go out with a boy, but it isn't all that serious. I am an anajetic person, as my mum says, I never get tired.

Really I don't think I'm a very nice person to know because I talk too much to people I know and yet I'm very shy to anyone else.

I get on well with people and like meeting them but I can't stand moany people, or people of our age or older who think themselves better than us. I can talk to people, but sometimes get tongue-tied with a nice boy.

I am a virgin and want to stay that way till I'm married. Sometimes when I go out with a boy I do get sort of spasms and do feel sexy, but I've found that I can control myself.

I haven't got a boy-friend although I do go out in a group with boys, but we don't often pair off.

The only thing is, I have to look after my brother and take him for a walk. This sometimes stops me from going out with boys because they want to go out at about 6 o'clock, but I have to look after my brother at that time, and this is every night I have to do this. I would like to get married when I am 19 years old.

I have no trouble with friends out of school, but in school I seem to be the odd one out. The girls in my form seem to think its not right for me not to go out with boys and not to wear make-up.

I have lots of friends out of school, but my best friend and I have known each other for nearly twelve years. She lives on the fifth floor of my block and we get on quite well together because we like the same things. I like boys, especially one that lives up the hill to me. In the holidays my friends and I go down the park or we go swimming. Sometimes I go out in the evenings but it is a bit boring at night round our way. We might go in my friend's house or just walk about and have a laugh and talk to some boys.

Comment

Despite much sophisticated bravado, on average only half a dozen girls in each form had boyfriends in the specific or sexual sense. I have no evidence that any were indulging in intercourse or even heavy petting, which of course does not prove that this does not go on in this age group. But my impression of the girls in each form of 30 is that only about half go out at all and of these, half go out with girls or in a mixed crowd and half have boyfriends. Very few indeed had serious boyfriends who lasted more than a few weeks and the ones who did appeared to regard them primarily as good companions and to have what was basically an asexual relationship. This would not of course be true for the fourth year and upwards.

Sparetime activities

At night I am allowed to go out but there is nowhere to go.

I like walking through the Park on a Summer's day.

I am allowed out when I want to which is not very often as there is not any clubs or dances where I live and you usually have to travel to get anywhere interesting.

I usually stay in and do my homework. Its a bit of a bore because I don't know anyone who lives near me–in the holidays its terrible.

I have a job on Saturdays, but as you are not going to show this to anyone, I can tell you because I am slightly under age.

I don't go out because there's nothing to do, only pictures.

I love strawberries and ice-cream, modern clothes, pop-music and boys. I hate spaghetti and school, going visiting my aunts, and doing homework.

I like ballet-dancing. My sister often says that I won't stick at it but I like it too much to give it up.

I go out most nights a week, on Wednesdays I go to evening class and on Fridays to a Youth Club.

I don't go out because I tend to worry about my homework and so I stay in and do it. I think we shouldn't have homework, especially over the weekend, because if you are going away you have got your homework to worry about, and not only that, we spend five days at school a week, writing and so they should give us a rest.

I like needlework, reading and listening to records. I like boys but my mum won't let me go out with them.

When I am not working or reading, I take dogs or babys for a walk with my friends, my favourite sport is swimming.

I have not got many interests because I do not have time for them. I like watching TV.

I like ice skating, needlework and dancing bot not going swimming. I like listening to pop records and I like meeting new friends of both sexes.

I love horse riding. I go to the stables every day.

My hobbies are reading, sleeping, going for walks with friends and having a laugh.

Comment

Most of the girls claim not to go out very much, and to spend most of their spare time watching television. Some appear to have time to go out every night, some are too busy doing homework. The most disturbing comments are those about the lack of amenities in the area. In some cases this is the rationalization of a desire not to face the world, but more often it is true. The other problem is the parental veto: some half a dozen girls in each form are not allowed to go out at all, not even with girlfriends. They may not have set about asking very determinedly; most are happy to accept this housebound state at this age, but if it continues into the fourth year it becomes a real problem for them.

Ambitions

When I leave school I would like to be a computer operator but I shall have to work hard for this.

I don't know what to do when I leave school. I am staying on but I dislike school.

I would like an intelligent and easy going husband, a bit like me in some ways, a couple of children and some animals.

My ambition was to become a vet, but that idea went down the drain when I found the studying that had to be done.

My ambition is to work with horses.

I haven't a clue what I want to be but I shall be glad when I leave.

I would not like to be very famous, but I would like to have a lot of money so I could buy the things I like and go to the places I want to go. I feel terribly tied down at school. I know my work is very important for my future but sometimes I feel like just giving up and going out to work. I would never do this but sometimes it is very tempting.

When I leave school I'd like to be an air hostess I think, but I keep changing my mind.

We want to emigrate to Canada, that is, us girls and mum, but my dad doesn't.

I do not know what I want to do when I leave school, but I want to stay on to the seventh year to take A levels if I can.

I did want to be a tipest but I am not brainey enough.

I really am set on being an actress when I leave school although my parents don't agree. I can see their point, insecurity and so on. But I would hate to be stuck in an office in front of a typewriter. I feel this would bore me. I would be willing to work very hard to achieve my ambition though it may seem only a childish dream.

Comment

Most of the girls did not know what they wanted to do when they left school, which is hardly surprising as they are only aged 13-14 years. I have not given a fully representative list of job choices here. Most girls said they didn't know. The rest listed some occupation in a straightforward way. Most suggestions were, in line with Thelma Veness' research, realistic and not particularly exciting or ambitious.[2] A few had unrealistic aims, particularly immigrants: aspiring doctors with no hope of O levels, would-be ballet dancers who were totally untrained and quite the wrong shape anyway. This category of child needs skilful handling. I want to come back to these particular problems in more detail when I discuss relationships with careers officers.

Adolescent moods and general comments

I hate my name and I don't know what I want to do when I leave school. I like horseriding and swimming but I am not good at either of these things. I don't like homework or injections. I also disslike school doctors and school medicals. I am fat and tall and I am not very good in sliming.

I have a quick temper. I am quiet and shy.

I have had a rotten past. I was in a home most of my younger years.

My trouble is that I have a quick temper and I don't mean to argue but I get so annoyed that I can't help it. I bite my nails when I'm reading a book or watching television, but mostly when I'm nervous.

I am fat and I know I am fat. I am very self-conscious in the presence of men. I hope I will grow out of it.

My sisters and I are always argueing because I have a quick temper and they keep teasing me.

I bite my nails through nervousness, despite efforts to stop. I have moods when I get shy but I can usually hold my own and I'm usually happy and friendly.

I dislike cheese, people who always get embarrassed, men who think girls should be feminine, girls who are so thick skinned that they don't believe you when you say you don't like them. I like most people, drink, school (more or less) money, and pop groups.

My moods change far too rapidly for my liking.

One thing I hate, really hate is the dentist. Even the mention of it I burst into tears.

I have hundreds of secrets, just small things, things that would seem silly if I told my family, but they mean a lot to me. I seem to day-dream a lot.

I bite my nails through nervousness. This has something to do with school. In holidays they begin to grow but as soon as I come back to school I can't stop.

Since I came to secondary school, I have changed very much. I used to be timid and shy but now I have come well out of my shell, but I think I'm not such a nice person as I used to be.

I don't believe in marriage.

I get shy in front of people very easily and they often think I'm quiet but once they've gone I'm alright and I'm my normal self.

Have you eny idears how I could look my age becous I am very small for my age.

I dislike overbearing people, snobs, spoilt children, talk backs—people who become your friend and then talk about you behind your back, sweets, white coffee, my mother sometimes, my sister most of the time, the neighbours, racialism, prejudice, war, history. I like everything not listed above, especially my mum when I don't dislike her.

Comment

Not all the girls commented on their moods—they were not specifically asked to do so. What is interesting about their comments is the number who expressed grave self-doubts, which were largely unjustified; those who worried about being fat were, at most, simply rather luscious and nubile. Those who claimed to have violent tempers appeared to be quiet and calm. Those who patently *were* fat and aggressive did not usually comment on this on paper: either the point was too sensitive to them or too obvious to me to need elaborating. Often these girls would come and talk about their appearance or their moods afterwards.

Again most of the quotations I give are not from girls with serious problems. Their comments show already a degree of insight and sense of perspective which is healthy enough. More serious are the cases where the girls cannot express their feelings at all or where the only feelings expressed are hostile and negative.

Group discussion of these points

Although I have taken this selection of comments from the girls' autobiographical notes, they are typical of the kind of remark made in the group discussions. Thus many of the more obvious points of teenage conflict are dealt with there and then, spontaneously by the group. One of the purposes of the group discussion is for members to perceive and accept that it is normal to be different: for example not all girls of 13 or 14 want to go out in the evenings and certainly not with boys, yet many of them worry about this. Adults too are sometimes guilty of making similar sweeping statements about what girls of 14 should or should not do: 'A girl of your age shouldn't go out with boys, should be in by eight o'clock.' 'A girl of your age should get out a bit more, learn to mix a bit.' What we have to remember is that chronological age is not as important as developmental stage. Girls who mature later, or more slowly, need reassurance to gain the strength not to feel that they should be doing the same as their peers to prove that they are 'normal'. The group with its widely different views helps to provide this reassurance, more effectively than any single adult can. Girls who feel isolated from their contemporaries, girls who feel they are the odd one out, girls who have nowhere to go in the evenings or no friends in their neighbourhood may realize with a great sense of relief just how common these feelings are. They may come to understand and to accept that people develop in different ways and at different rates and gain some sense of their individual worth and values.

Sometimes it is easier for the girls to discuss someone else's problem. The counsellor might make up a problem like this: 'Janet was nearly 14. She didn't have any boyfriends and the other girls sometimes laughed at her. But really she wasn't interested in boys; she much preferred to stay in or if she did go out, to be with her best girlfriend. All the same, she began to worry about being the odd one out. What should she do?' The counsellor does not say. The girls themselves argue, suggest, discuss, at the same time gaining reassurance and developing a less narrow view of their friends. This is much more effective than a statement from the counsellor. It usually matters more to a girl what her friends think of her than what adults think.

Another common dilemma is illustrated by this example: 'Pauline's mother would not let her go out with boys even though she was nearly 14. Pauline didn't think it was fair. She was however allowed to go to a youth club once a week provided she was in by nine o'clock. One day a boy she particularly liked asked her to go to the pictures. Her friend Anna suggested she pretended to her mother that she was going out with her. What should Pauline do?'

Again the counsellor does not give the answer. There isn't an answer and it is far more valuable for the girls to argue this out among themselves. There are usually a few girls in each group who consider it quite logical to deceive one's parents in a case like this if the parents are not sufficiently confident to give permission and if the child feels that she can take full responsibility. Usually the problem is that the girls have not had the courage to discuss the issue with their parents and are assuming a negative reply. Or they ask permission for something unacceptable like going to see an X film, are firmly told 'No' and then take it that they will never be allowed to go anywhere. We may spend some time discussing how to set about this question of getting permission to go out for the first time. The more experienced girls help the others; mostly it is a question of gaining enough confidence to bring the matter to a head. Some girls are not sufficiently secure in their relationship with their parents to take a stand on any issue yet eventually this is what they will have to do to gain any measure of independence. Some ask for independence but are frightened of actually having any, which is why they ask hesitantly and then blame their parents for the negative reply which has saved them from facing the dangers of freedom. Sometimes there *is* a genuine problem here: parents who will not let their daughters out of the house at all, sometimes immigrants, sometimes over-possessive parents who do not want their children to grow up. I have come across several girls who pretended they did not *want* to go out rather than admit to their friends that their parents would not let them. These girls have been guarded in the group but have come afterwards to talk in private about their dilemma.

There is no doubt that parents sometimes are a real problem: too rigid parental control, or none, or inconsistencies. Sometimes the parents are insecure in their own relationships or their own social situation. Marital disharmony, financial worries, overcrowding, ill health, loss of job or status, mental breakdown—all these factors make for strain in a family. Sometimes a child with the most difficult home situation manages to remain resilient and cheerful, indeed may grow in strength and understanding through this adverse experience. Sometimes a child may get the family situation out of perspective and blame herself for all the pain and anxiety that surround her. Such a child can be helped, sometimes through generalized group discussion, to see that the way other people treat us sometimes has nothing to do with our actual behaviour and response but is more a reflection of their own emotional needs. If a child can come to understand a difficult situation in her family she can often learn to tolerate it or even help to ease it.

We must not however expect young people to be too tolerant. A girl with a handicapped brother or an over-tired working mother or a physical disability of her own may appear to cope with an astonishing degree of forbearance and responsibility. Often these girls are under considerable strain and need the counsellor's help to gather for themselves the strength to communicate some consideration of their own point of view and needs to the rest of the family. In the group, individuals are not encouraged to express these sorts of personal problems at any length; they may work out their own answer through group discussion or they may come later for individual counselling.

Questions about sex

This glimpse of the adolescent world would not be complete without some consideration of the girls' attitudes towards sex. As I have already explained, at least one of the group discussions is devoted to questions about sex and other sessions may be devoted to discussions about allied social problems. Although there is not a syllabus to be covered we find from experience that the same topics inevitably arise. The girls have had instruction about human reproduction in the first year and are well acquainted with the facts of life, though some have forgotten some things, perhaps because they were too young to take it all in at the time.

They therefore usually welcome the chance to go over again the topics of menstruation, intercourse and childbirth and to have the opportunity to ask supplementary questions. They are still often worried about old wives' tales or confused about veiled allusions they have heard to such things as VD, the Pill, Durex, homosexuality, perversion. They cannot escape reading about these matters in newspapers or hearing about them in television plays and discussions but it is sometimes hard for them to piece together what they hear and see in such an oblique manner. The object of talking about it all is not to equip them with sophisticated know-how, but to remove from these topics any aura of furtive secrecy and provocative mystery, to replace worry with reassurance, fantasy with fact. It is doubtful whether the girls remember what they are told in any detail.

The questions asked about sex vary tremendously in maturity, sophistication and purpose. Some are clearly asked simply to shock the counsellor and see if she is really trustworthy and permissive as she says. Many give the impression of a degree of sexual experience way beyond the norm for such young girls: in most cases I am sure this is either because of bravado (which seems to exist among girls as well as boys) or unfortunate phrasing. However I think it is important for adults to realize the kind of questions young adolescents ask about sex. I also think it important that those who are training to answer these questions should experience something of the directness of the teenage approach. Children rarely ask textbook questions requiring textbook answers, as you will see from the examples of questions asked. When the questions are factual they are answered factually; when they are a matter of opinion or subjects for discussion they are put before the group. You might like to think about how you would answer them.

Questions about menstruation/puberty

Is it wise for girls of our age to use sanitary towels like Tampax? If not, why? If it is wise could you advise us a kind to use? What age should we start to use them at?
If a girl is worried about not starting her periods, at what age should she consult her doctor?
When you have got your period, why don't you feel well?
Why are some people flat, and some have a good figure?
If a girl misses her periods two or three months, what should she do? Should she worry although she wasn't playing about with boys?
How do you improve your bust?
Should you get your hair wet when having periods?
Is it safe to go swimming while your period is on?
Should your boyfriend know when you've started, and if he did, what do you think he would do?

Questions about boys

Explain masturbation and is it wrong?
Could you explain what circumcision is?
Why do boys get frustrated?
Is it true that every kiss takes three minutes off your life?
If a boy comes near you when you are undressed can you become pregnant?
Why does a boy like you holding his private?
What is the average age for a boy to have an erection?
Why do boys and men go on the horn?
Why is it that girls are raped a lot and boys are rarely raped?
Can you tell whether a man is clean or has got VD?

Virginity

Is it possible to lose your virginity without actually having sexual intercourse? Excluding riding etc.
Can you lose your virginity through horse riding etc? How can you

tell if you have and what happens if you do?
Is it possible for a doctor to tell whether you are a virgin or not?
Why are people shocked when you say you're not a virgin? Because this is modern times and also why do boys take a nasty attitude and call you names when mostly they are boys of our own age?
What is breaking-in please?
Can your husband tell if you have had sexual intercourse before marriage?
If you've had sexual intercourse and you haven't had a baby are you still a virgin?
Why does it hurt when a boy breaks you in?
If a schoolboard or Welfare Officer found out she wasn't a virgin, would she be put in ball stalls *(sic)*?
Is it true about the medical you have in the fourth year that they look and see if you've been broken in? And do they do anything about it, eg inform parents?

Questions about behaviour with boys

Is petting wrong at our age?
What's the meaning of French kisses?
Why do boys have to break you in?
At what age do you think a girl should be broken in?
Does a boy go after you for what you have got or is it because he likes you or loves you?
Should you let boys do anything they want to? If not, what should you let them do and what shouldn't you let them do?
If you go out with a boy for the first time and he starts getting dirty and asks you to go steady, should you continue the relationship if you like him a lot?
Should you let a boy stroke your breasts?
Can love bites lead to trouble?
How do you control a boy with wandering hands?
Why does a boy lick your vagina?
Do you think it is right that a girl should suck a boy's prick?
If a boy is kissing you and he touches your body, should you walk off or let him do it?

Questions about childbirth

What is it like to be pregnant?
Is it dangerous to have sexual intercourse while you are pregnant?
What would happen if a girl became pregnant before she was 16 years old?
What is a miscarriage?
Can you explain a Caesarian operation?
Why do some women not know when they are pregnant?

Does it hurt very much when the baby comes out?
What do they mean by 'Oh, it was an accident' as if they didn't know she was pregnant?
How would you explain to your parents that you were having a baby?
Can you tell us about breaking the waters?
How are twins formed?
Is it dangerous to have an abortion?
Can you tell us about the afterbirth?
When a woman is sterilized does she still have periods?
If a girl is under 21 and is not married and is pregnant, and the mother of the girl wants her to get rid of the baby and the girl doesn't, can she still keep the child?
If a girl had a baby under 16 would the father of the baby go to court?
How are abortions performed? What are the dangers of such an operation?

Questions about intercourse

Is it right that newly-married couples have a sexual intercourse on their first night of marriage?
Do you have intercourse on your stomach or on your side?
Does it hurt to have intercourse?
How many positions can you have intercourse in?
Can you have intercourse while you are having your monthly period?
What happens to the semen that has not fertilized an egg but remains in the vagina?
How long does an intercourse last?
Would anything happen if you slept with your relation (eg brother)?
Can a man give a woman a baby at any age or time?
Is it true that when you have a sexual intercourse for the first time, that there is pain and loss of blood?
When you have intercourse do you have it on your periods or off?
When should you have intercourse, for how long and does it hurt?
How do you feel after you have had intercourse?
Is it safe to be intimate before marriage if you take precautions?

Questions about birth control

What is Durex?
How does the Pill work?
Are contraceptives dangerous?
Can you be sure not to have a baby when the boy uses Durex?
What is a diaphragm?

Questions about VD

Is it possible to catch VD by kissing if the boy is infected?
Do you only get VD when you have it away with other men, or when you just have it with one person? Because someone I know had VD and she only had it with one person.
What is VD really?
Why do we get discharge?
Can you get VD round the mouth through kissing many boys?
How do you get VD and how to you get rid of it?

Questions about homosexuality and perversion

Could you explain what is a pervert?
Why do homosexuals prefer men to the opposite sex as it is sickening and unnatural?
What does it mean when you read in the papers that a girl has been sexually assaulted?
What is a pansy?
What's the difference between being raped and being seduced?
What are homosexual practices?
Why are some women attracted to other women?

General questions asked

Is sex before marriage wrong?
Is it wrong to be a prostitute?
Why do mothers try to change the subject when their children ask them questions about boys, sex and the body?
Why do girls fall in love with pop stars and dream about them when they haven't the nearest chance of getting to know them?
Why do some parents have a favourite son or daughter if they have about three or four kids?
Why do some people make out sex to be wrong, even if you are married, when you have a baby?
Why do parents try to stop you growing up quicker (by wearing make-up and grown-up clothes) when at our age, 14, they were old enough to go out to work?
Do you think parents should open their daughters' letters or listen to their phone calls?
What is meant by trial marriage?
Should a girl go on holiday with a boy without parents?
I feel much more at home asking questions on sex and discussing it with my boyfriend than with anybody else as I can really face him and ask him at the same time. Is this right?

Comment

You may well be asking yourself at this point whether you really think girls of 13-14 years should be allowed to ask questions like this and moreover be given answers to them. You may feel that some of these questions are for much older children or possibly better not asked at all. But the point is that they *have* been asked by young adolescents. They were not prompted; they arose spontaneously. Just a few have been cooked up to shock or provoke, but most are genuine. I am assured by colleagues who work with boys that boys' questions are similar. Answering the questions, even questions of fact, is a delicate and skilled task. If the counsellor is worried for example about shocking the unsophisticated for the sake of explaining to the sophisticated few, this very anxiety will be conveyed in the answers. The counsellor needs a calmness, a lightness of touch, a sense of humour, an ability to talk about intimate matters without making them provocative and salacious or sweeping them under the carpet. It is not easy and this is why it is important for any teacher undertaking this work to be carefully selected, trained and supervised. The Marriage Guidance Council runs summer schools to help teachers interested in this work. Some counties, such as Gloucestershire and Wiltshire, have their own training schemes for education in personal relationships. What is potentially damaging or distressing about this kind of work is not the content of the group discussion so much as the way the subjects are handled. The feelings and attitudes behind what is being said are what will make the discussion responsible and fruitful, or otherwise. The more the girls themselves, rather than the counsellor, lead the discussion, the more they are likely to think and to take responsibility for themselves.

In fact it is debatable whether it is a good idea to ask for written questions at all even though there may always be a few questions which are important to ask but too difficult for the individual to voice. Writing down questions makes for a degree of impersonality which may reduce embarrassment but does I think provoke more test questions. Wherever possible we get the girls to put their questions in person. This gives the counsellor an opportunity to check whether she understands the questions, and it often leads to more discussion (rather than just question and answer) and more responsible discussion at that.

In answering the questions about sex it is often more rewarding for the counsellor to group together questions say about menstruation and to review the whole topic, taking care to answer, not avoid, the original question. Similarly questions about intercourse, childbirth, boys' sexual behaviour should be faced squarely. One question answered in isolation can create an odd, one-sided impression and may be better treated as part of a whole.

In fact the amount of time we spend on this part of the discussion is very little—one session, two at most. Thus most subjects are touched on superficially. The girls enjoy talking about marriage, how they are going to bring up their children, whether they want to plan their families or work when they have children. Sometimes the discussion turns to issues such as racial prejudice or social injustice, or to a group problem such as how to handle a troublemaker within the form

What girls are most interested in discussing are the problems which come within their own range of experience. The main part of the discussion concerns the normal problems of adolescence: worries about menstruation and moodiness, conflicts with parents about going out and having boyfriends, anxieties over appearance or about the way to behave in a new situation, problems of having nowhere to go in the evenings and no friends in their neighbourhood. Through talking together the girls can realize with relief just how common these problems are. They can realize that other people too have problem parents, terrible brothers and sisters, nagging grandparents. Through their common human predicament they are able to gain a sense of perspective, become more tolerant and take their problems less personally. If by the end of the group discussions they are still insecure or worried about anything they have the opportunity of talking further in an individual interview. Sometimes they have already indicated their problem in the group or in their autobiographical note. It is against this background of general comment from girls who did not have serious problems that I want now to discuss the comments made by those particular girls who needed individual counselling.

References

1. J. Hemming *Problems of Adolescent Girls* (Heinemann 1967)
2. T. Veness *School Leavers: Their Aspirations and Expectations* (Methuen 1962)

Chapter 7

Individuals

In this chapter I give examples of problems faced by adolescent girls and brought to the counsellor in school. Teachers often ask me whether boys' problems are any different, or whether it matters if the counsellor is a man or a woman. My discussions with counsellors who see boys confirm that the nature of adolescent boys' problems is similar to girls': to do with relationships with their nearest and dearest, with the search for identity and role and with the quest for independence and freedom without total loss of family support. Boys may be more overtly aggressive than girls, they may also seek to hide their tender feelings in the mistaken idea that these detract from their masculinity. But basically their problems will be similar to girls' with differences more in emphasis.

The sex of the counsellor seems to me not to matter, provided the counsellor is not exploiting the interview to satisfy his sexual needs (ie his need to be admired by the opposite sex, his need to be reassured that he is attractive, his need to form a dependent relationship). Even with counsellor and client of the same sex, similar problems may be encountered if the counsellor has not come to terms with his own needs or is not aware of the ways he and his client are interacting. The only time the sex of the counsellor might be important is when the client needs to relate to a father-figure rather than a mother-figure or vice versa. If a school has more than one counsellor it might well decide to have one male and one female counsellor and to let the students select which they prefer. But if there is no choice, no matter. Much more important than the sex of the counsellor are his counselling skills and the quality of the relationship he forms with his client.

The examples I give in this and the succeeding chapter are intended simply to illustrate the *types* of problems that a counsellor may come across and to indicate what I thought was the counsellor's role. I have grouped problems with a similar flavour together though no two problems are identical. I have commented briefly on each group of examples at the end of each section. But my intention, with the examples and with the comment, is to spell out 'the answer' as little as possible. Apart from the fact that interpretations vary and that there certainly isn't *an* answer, I prefer to leave room for my readers to think about each case. If in my efforts to make my points clear I have over-simplified or become dogmatic, I apologize. Were this book meant to teach counselling techniques, then my approach would be different. This book is meant as a statement of problems rather than a manual of answers.

I must also remind you that I have of course changed all the names and much of the detail in the examples I quote, though the nature of the problems remains as it was in real life.

Communication

Jennifer (14)

'I have parents and sisters with whom I do not get on. My mother often worries me and is extremely cross with me continually. I have few friends out of home as I do not make friends easily. My mother is strict about what I do and has a firm hand in what I wear. I am not allowed to wear make-up or short skirts. I help a lot in the house and have hardly any time for myself. I hardly ever have time to watch television or go out.'

Jennifer felt sufficiently strongly about her situation to write about her life in these terms. The first interview with her confirmed the impression given by her note—namely that she felt a lack of positive regard from her nearest and dearest, she lacked confidence in herself, she was anxious, she bit her nails. At school she was no problem. Her work and behaviour gave no cause for complaint, though her form teacher observed that she had few friends. Her lack of self-confidence did in fact make her manner tense. Her negative attitudes undoubtedly detracted from her desirability as a companion. She needed to gain enough self-confidence to communicate her feelings to her mother, to assert her independence from her mother's rigid control at least in some small measure and to learn to relate better to her peers.

Her mother had a full-time job from which she returned tired and tense. Despite Jennifer's protestations it became clear that she really did enjoy the responsibility she took for preparing the evening meal and helping generally. What she could not tolerate was the fact that her efforts did not seem to be appreciated. True she was given pocket money in exchange for her help but frequently her efforts at cooking and cleaning would be criticized by both her parents. Mother in particular appeared to Jennifer to be moody and unjustifiably critical at times. Jennifer also felt jealous and resentful of an older sister who was seriously ill and therefore escaped household chores and received a lot of extra mothering.

It seemed to me that the problem was largely one of communication. Jennifer's mother was probably not aware of the effect her behaviour and attitudes were having on Jennifer, and Jennifer lacked sufficient confidence to air her grievances, simply storing them up into a grudge.

At various stages we discussed the possibility of my seeing the mother. This Jennifer decided against, I think not so much because she felt it was *her* job to do this, but because she was ambivalent towards her mother and afraid of the responsibility of replacing her mother's control with her own. Thus she allowed the unhappy home situation to continue for half a term before she felt sufficient confidence to bring matters to a head. She wanted to grow up, but not too quickly, and a small measure of autonomy was all that was needed to boost her self-esteem. Most important of all to her was to have her mother's affection and appreciation instead of her payment and criticism. It was interesting that despite the hostility expressed towards her mother initially she wanted to be a secretary like her mother.

One week Jennifer arrived very elated to report that she had had a 'big row' with her mother during which she had explained her feelings and stated that she was going out on certain evenings to do voluntary community work. She also decided to wear make-up. From this moment her attitude towards her mother changed: she expressed admiration for the way her mother coped with a job *and* a home. She also became more tolerant of her father and her sister. Her whole appearance began to alter: she stood well instead of hunched, her eyes sparkled beneath their make-up (worn even to school), she stopped biting her nails and her hair shone.

She came to see me for a few more weeks during which she reported that her mother now trusted her in the kitchen and had praised her cooking. She expressed sympathy for her sister's illness and need for attention. She began to talk of her career plans. She felt less tired and was enjoying life more. At this stage we decided to discontinue counselling with the understanding that Jennifer could always come back if this happier state of affairs did not continue. Jennifer did not expect to live happily ever after but she had made a good first step towards helping herself. Her form teacher confirmed that Jennifer had a more relaxed and confident approach to life.

Louise (16)

Louise came back to see me in the fifth year. She was an only child living in a household of adults who included not only her parents but also her maternal grandmother; her father's stepmother also visited frequently. Because of this environment Louise had taken on the attitudes and standards of an older generation. She was extremely conscientious and law-abiding. She felt her form mates regarded her as 'goody-goody' and old-fashioned. She did not have any boy-friends nor did she feel she had much hope of getting any.

But this was not her immediate problem. Her problem was rather that in spite of her 'goodness' she was not very well regarded by her peers; this began to throw doubts in her mind as to the virtues of being 'good'. Yet, at the same time she was frightened and horrified at facing the imperfections and 'bad thoughts' both within herself and her family.

She referred herself for counselling at this stage because she was beginning to realize that neither she nor her family was perfect. She began to feel the atmosphere at home claustrophobic. Although she did many good community deeds, she felt she was not getting any fun out of life. She asked for more independence at home but with so many adults to organize, discuss and control her life she found it difficult to gain any.

She began to ventilate her feelings, including her bad feelings, which I accepted without being shocked as normal reaction in her situation and at her age. One day she said she was going to let her hair down and when I looked at her I saw that she had done just this, literally. It was very important for her to begin to release her total self instead of only letting out the 'good' and controlling the 'bad'. Again she did not want me to see her parents, although it took a half term of counselling before she had gained sufficient freedom in herself to assert herself at home. The final straw came when she had to give up her room to yet another relative who was coming to stay. At last she had the courage to express herself to her family, who as a result accorded her the respect and adult status she desired and gave her back her room. She made only a small step forward; she was then happy to return to the security of the family network. But in terms of self-assertion and self-acceptance she had an important beginning.

Geraldine (13)

Geraldine's grandfather was getting her down. There was nothing anyone could do about it. The family doctor was already trying to find an old people's home for him though Geraldine's mother was resisting. Mother was clearly carrying a great deal of strain. It seemed to me that she was probably not aware how much Geraldine and her sister were suffering from the side effects of grandfather's nagging, and mother's preoccupation with his problems at the expense of everyone else's.

Geraldine decided to talk to her mother about how she felt instead of suffering and building up resentment. This seemed to improve communications between mother and daughter and help mother to weigh her various duties more rationally. For example, shortly after, mother at last took up the offer of the social services that they should look after grandfather while mother took a holiday. For the first time for years the parents and children took a holiday without grandfather in tow.

Betty (14)

'I have three sisters aged 3, 11 and 16 years. I argue a lot with the two eldest. My eldest sister goes out a lot to clubs and shows, which makes me quite jealous, of course, she won't let me go, so this causes arguments. My eldest sister is very modern and tries to help me a lot but being quite fat I can't get modern clothes to fit me. I get on with my parents alright now and again, although I don't think they like me as much as the others, because I get blamed for everything, I am quite unhappy at home and at school. I really hate school. I have no boyfriends though I would like one.'

Betty described herself as the family scapegoat, the odd one out, the only fat one, the one who took the blame for everything. It seemed unlikely to me that the actual situation was quite as bas as this but this was how it seemed to Betty, which is what mattered. Her dissatisfaction with school reflected the low opinion she had come to have of herself; she was becoming negative and apathetic and was also eating too much in spite of her intention to slim. Our objectives were therefore to increase her self-respect through the relationship with the counsellor, to help her to communicate with her family her needs and feelings and to help her understand better the pressures within the family as a whole.

The jealousy between the sisters and their rivalry for the parents' attention is both real and normal enough with children of these ages. But one factor that contributed a great deal to Betty's self-destructive attitude was the guilt she felt through having dropped her baby sister out of the pram when the baby was six months old. Thus her 11-year-old sister and her 16-year-old sister were able to curry parental favour by taking out the youngest child. Betty was not allowed to do this because she was not regarded as trustworthy and she did not trust herself.

Because of her self-deprecatory attitude, she brought upon herself the deprecation of the rest of the family and thus became a ready-made vehicle for many of their bad feelings. As a result she became resentful, sullen and fat. How to break the vicious circle?

Shortly after counselling began Betty decided to ask for some clothes. Apart from her school uniform she had no smart clothes. This was one reason she did not go out more; she often turned down invitations rather than have to appear in school uniform. To her surprise her mother supported the idea of more clothes. Betty had misjudged her mother's attitude towards her. Mother took a stand on this, which made Betty appreciate her mother more and feel that her mother did care about her after all.

Unfortunately there *was* no spare money in the family, as father was under considerable strain, financial and emotional, because he was having to support a relative of his. Thus Betty realized that her father *did* care about her and *did* want her to look pretty but that money was tight for other reasons. This increased her respect for her father. Two-way communication with her parents became re-established. They bought her a dress in spite of hard times, which provided just that bit of extra attention she needed to feel on the same footing as her sisters.

What happened in school? Betty became more cheerful and confident. She was elected form spokesman on a school matter, which increased her self-confidence enormously. She took a leading part in helping another girl in the form. She finally admitted to me that her older sister also had serious problems, which is probably why she had so much attention from her parents.

Thus she realized that she was not, as she had thought, the weakest member of the family but one of the strongest. She continued to play a supportive role within her family but this time without being destroyed by her own self-doubts or being taken for granted by others.

Pamela (13)

Pamela was the oldest in a family of six children. Her mother had divorced when she was a baby, remarried when she was five. Pamela had adjusted reasonably well to all this. She said that her problem was simply that with so many younger brothers and sisters, she found it difficult to get on with her homework. One young brother (seven) in particular teased her and got on her nerves a great deal. She could not work in her room because there was no fire. The problem may in fact have been much deeper than this, but this is the level at which Pamela expressed it.

It seems incredible to me that she should not have discussed this with her parents or even with her form tutor. It is not a particularly confidential or sensitive matter. But she had not. After seeing me she did talk to her mother, who immediately got her an electric fire while her stepfather had a chat with the brother, who then became less of a nuisance. It was a simple matter, though it may have helped to serve complicated needs. It is not however untypical of the kind of problem which a girl of this age puts up with rather than dare to ask her parents about.

COMMENT. In these first examples there was nothing to be 'done'. It was far more constructive for the girls to communicate their needs to their parents than for me to step in on their behalf. The basic problem was internal rather than external; the actual situations in which these girls lived were not intolerable, and in any case there was no changing them. What had gone wrong, in each case, was the individual child's perception of the situation. Her inability to communicate her needs and feelings to her parents and siblings had turned them against her. At the same time she herself became a victim of destructive self-doubts and self-pity. Communicating with the counsellor was the first step towards communicating with her parents. Once she had done this, she began to see her life in better perspective.

Confidentiality

Brenda (13)

Brenda referred herself after third year groups with a secret she had shared with no one. Her note was ordinary enough; she herself was a pleasant and reliable child. She asked for an appointment and then in the first interview began to explain what was troubling her. As far as she could make out, her sister had had an illegitimate baby when Brenda was 11. The problem was that no one in the family had ever talked to her about this, presumably because they thought she was too young at the time to know about such things without getting upset.

Unfortunately *not* knowing was making her more upset. Her sister came to visit every few weeks but there was this taboo topic of conversation between them. Furthermore her own developing sexual feelings made her feel frightened and ambivalent both about what had happened to her sister and what might happen to her. She was very fond of her sister but always upset after seeing her. Her parents were strict, both over 50. Brenda found it difficult to talk to them about sex or indeed any of her feelings.

Her need to talk about her problem was great yet she could not talk to her form tutor about it because she did not want to let her family down. Through talking to the counsellor she began to express her feelings and gain sufficient confidence to get her family to tell her the whole story. This served the double function of relieving her worries and according her more adult status. Her case provides a clear example of a problem in which the counsellor's outside role and the confidential basis of the relationship with her were very important.

Josephine (14)

'I like going out in the evenings with my friend. I am shy when I'm with boys and have at present no boyfriend. I have an older brother. A couple of months ago he went through a stage of being very catty towards me. I think he went through this stage because before this he had tried petting me which I did not like and so I threatened to tell mum and dad. I would never have dreamed of doing this because I knew I would get into trouble as well. Also I did not think it right to tell them.'

She only came to see me once. She needed to tell someone 'safe' all about it. This helped her face her own guilty feelings. She seemed to have coped with the incident at the time; it was all over and there was nothing to be done about it that would have been constructive. She was not asking for help with her own sexual development and she did not want the matter to go any further. She knew she could come back later if she wanted. We left it at that.

Veronica (14)

'I have a boyfriend living some way away, so I only see him at weekends at the moment, though when he gets his motorbike I shall see him more frequently. He is studying for his A levels. My mother does not agree with my going out with him although she puts up with it. My father wants me to stay on for A levels.'

Veronica was a mature-looking girl who could pass for 16-17 years although she was only 14. She had been in love with her boyfriend for over a year. Every Saturday he came to spend the day at her house. On Sundays his parents would leave them alone in their house. What was worrying her was the strength of her own sexual feelings. She was sincere and steady in her love for him; she was reaching the point where she was finding heavy petting very frustrating and she was wanting to go on to have intercourse.

The fact that she wanted to talk to me about it first shows that in part at least she was worried and in doubt about what she should do. We talked it over for several weeks. I reminded her about the age of consent and answered several factual questions as well as discussing the possible psychological, social and legal results of her proposed action. During the discussion it emerged that she had a poor relationship with her parents who seemed to take little real interest or to realize remotely what she was doing: 'Had a good day, dear? Fine.'

Veronica herself had little time for girls of her own age; she did not seem to be able to widen her own interests. Thus all her need for love, affection and security was going into this one boy. He was not pressing her to go any further. Her battle was with her own desires. She left me very thoughtfully, a little more aware of the complicated forces which were driving her. The whole discussion had been confidential: without this safeguard I do not think she would have talked at all. She did not want me to communicate with her parents; I hope she began to do so herself. She knew she could get contraceptive advice and counselling, despite her youth, through a clinic nearby. She knew that she could come back to see me any time she wanted.

She came back six months later to tell me that after a lot of discussion she and her boyfriend had decided to break off their relationship as they felt it was getting too intense. During the holidays she had met someone else; though it had not lasted, it had made her think. By the next term the other girls in the form had grown up a bit and she found that she had more in common with them than she had thought.

Beth (13)

'I go swimming regularly in London. This causes concern at home. It is a long way away and my parents don't like me getting too involved with the attendants there as I do.'

She was worried about it too: she found the attendants devastatingly attractive, especially the one who was already engaged. Although basically she had a good relationship with her parents she found it difficult to discuss this problem with them as their attitude was tinged with disapproval from the start. She worked out her own answer through talking to someone who could allow her the freedom to express her own doubts without loss of face.

COMMENT. These girls all had problems which they needed to talk over with an adult, but which they could only share with an adult they could trust absolutely. Any precipitate action by the counsellor, any condemnation would have stopped them talking. Not that the counsellor condoned: we must not equate an accepting adult with a consenting adult. But if the counsellor cannot accept the 'bad' in each child the child will continue to cover over her real problem. For various reasons, these were problems that the girls found difficult to discuss with their parents or form tutor. The counsellor's role as an outsider who could be trusted with confidential information was important.

A friendly adult

Marion (13)

'When I was young my mother and I lived with my grandparents. I was sent to nursery school until I was five. At the age of six my mother married a man who adopted me as his daughter. He is now my father. He is very good and kind to me and I would not have anyone else in the world. My mother is happy with him also. I have no brothers or sisters.'

Nevertheless soon after she wrote this Marion came back to see me, filled with a desire to see her real father, from whom her mother had separated when Marion was very young. She realized that this might be an upsetting or disappointing experience, but her need to establish her true identity was great. She talked to her parents about it. They understood her very well; finally they told her the whole story of her early life; her grandmother also joined in and produced photos of her real father.

These revelations did in fact upset the happy balance of Marion's family for a while. She needed me to talk to about her sudden anger and resentment with her mother. She worked through her mixed feelings eventually. I'm not sure that she had been quite ready for the whole truth but the search for identity is certainly strong and overwhelming at this stage.

Donna (14)

Donna was worried about being fat. She *was* a little plump. Her current friends constantly teased her, particularly in mixed company, which completely undermined her confidence. She was interested in boys but had no hope of getting a boyfriend in these conditions. She told me all about it. She then decided to join a new youth club. She found her new friends accepted her as a lively and amusing companion. She found that boys did like her after all. She was able to withstand her old friends' criticisms, which began to fall off when they discovered they had little effect.

Frances (18)

Frances was referred to the counsellor by the staff in her seventh year. She was feeling very depressed and attributed this to her father's moodiness. She talked a lot about her father's moods, then went on to say why she thought he was like this. A week later she returned to say she had much greater sympathy for her father; they had begun to talk more and she felt generally less tense and worried.

It seemed too good to be true to me but there is no judging the effects of even one counselling session if it comes at an appropriate moment. Frances was intelligent and already showed insight. The counselling interview may have served to crystallize her thoughts and to focus them for once on her father's needs as opposed to her own. Having started on a new train of thought she may well have gone on following it throughout the week or she may have just covered over her difficulties again. Who knows?

Tao-Tao (13)

'I really have a terrible time in here because of the language and no friends. I only learnt English less than two years.

'In my country I had a few friends but they are very nice so I didn't think that I wish more friends. I didn't know friends are most important thing in my life. I understand perfectly now why they are important. I want friends to invite to my house. But I can't because the way of living is completely different. Studying is no matter, language is no matter if I learn it, but I am a lonely girl. I don't think

I can make friend by myself, never. I am a terribly shy girl.'

Tao-Tao came from the Far East during the second year. She was highly intelligent but shy by nature—not just because of language difficulties. She was proud too and did not communicate her loneliness to her form tutor. To me she expressed, in her halting English, some of her worries. Going to boarding school back home would not help her, because she now preferred the freedom (eg to have boyfriends) of the Western culture. My role was simply to befriend her until she found herself.

By the end of the next term she had made several friends and was feeling much happier.

Audry (15)

Audry, an attractive, black girl, came back in the fourth year to complain that her father was too strict: he didn't trust her. I asked her whether she *was* trustworthy. It rather surprised her to realize that she was not. It dawned on her that this was perhaps why her father did not trust her. She decided to be straight with him.

She came back a month later to say he now let her go out to the Palais de Danse once a week provided she was in by eleven o'clock. She had been doing this for ages, pretending she had been going to see a cousin. She said she felt much better now that her father knew where she really was; he had been much pleasanter once he realized she could cope with the young men she met.

Alethea (13)

Alethea had Greek-Cypriot parents who never gave her a chance to prove that she was trustworthy. It was really a cultural problem. 'I've got a feeling that my parents are going to choose my husband as most Cypriots do, but I despise this idea and want to find my own husband.'

When I saw her she was simply wanting to be allowed out occasionally. She did not want me to talk to her parents as 'that would only make them cross; they wouldn't change at all.' As she was still young at the time she decided to bear her problem a little longer. She felt better for having talked it over. The really testing time for someone caught in the cultural crossfire like this is when she is 16. If she does not want to marry someone of her father's choice or be relegated to the kitchen sink but prefers to complete her education, choose her own job and husband, then real conflict begins. We have a lot of girls with similar problems: some Greek-Cypriots, some Indians, some Pakistanis.

COMMENT. These girls were not really asking for me to do anything, not even help them communicate better with their parents. They just wanted to talk to an adult outside the family. What they had to say was not confidential in the sense of being an explosive secret but it was private and they wanted it to be treated with respect and privacy. They needed the relationship with the counsellor to help them through a difficult but transitory stage in their lives.

Support

Anita (14)

Anita is a good example of a girl whose problem was not what it seemed at first. She referred herself in the first place because her sister-in-law was about to have a baby and this was worrying her. But it was not as simple as this. She lived with her sister-in-law to help look after the first baby. This made her feel insecure about her mother, whom she only saw at weekends. Her mother worked all the week, so she reckoned she would not see much of her even if she were at home. But living with her brother and his wife in these particular circumstances made her aware of her own sexual feelings, which both fascinated and repulsed her. She felt that if she went out with boys she would get a bad reputation or become pregnant. She was particularly sensitive about what other people might say about her.

This feeling went back to an accident when she was eight when a friend of hers was killed. She felt in some way responsible and thought other people had held this against her. In fact it was not in any way her fault. When she had managed to talk about this she became less worried about her current reputation.

It took her several weeks to pluck up courage to tell me about this incident. At that stage I had begun to think that her problems were not all that serious. This shows the danger of the counsellor's judging that there are no 'real' problems and not allowing the client time to come to the point. It was not the only point in this case but it was important to Anita to come to it. Once she had expressed her guilty secret she became more secure generally.

Soon after this her sister-in-law's baby was born. Anita did not, as she imagined she would, have to cope with the two-year-old child during the confinement and she went to live back at home. Her father then went into hospital for an operation but this did not worry her unduly. She was already more confident, having regained her mother and survived the birth of her nephew. She then found a steady boyfriend, who despite her previous fears, behaved in a very non-threatening way. He was 16, but she reckoned young and small for his age. Her fears about sex were allayed; she had the security of a good friend without any complications. She was thus much more able to face the grown-up world realistically. Most of her problems had sorted themselves out through various turns of events but I think it was important to her to be able to express her worst fears about herself and about sex while she was in such an insecure developmental stage. Supportive counselling was in fact just what she needed.

Angela (15)

Angela had gone to live in a children's home at the age of four when her parents divorced. When she was eight her mother remarried and took her back. Angela liked her stepfather and new brother but clearly was ambivalent about her mother, who was often ill and irritable. She came to see me because she felt her parents were exploiting her by using her in their shop. However it became clear that this was not really the problem. In fact she enjoyed working in the shop. She came to see me to chat about life, her feelings, her fears. She came, sporadically and spontaneously, until she left school at the end of the fourth year. There was nothing to be done about her; she was not in any dilemma about what she should do. She just needed more mothering than her real mother was able to provide at this stage. The relationship with the counsellor helped her to face the vicissitudes of her life more cheerfully and rationally.

Rachel (15)

Rachel had one older brother and three younger brothers. Her problem was in her relationship with her mother, who had just started a teacher training course. All the children were at school all day; father was co-operative and helpful with the domestic chores. Rachel, as the only girl, was expected to help a lot; the boys did relatively little.

Rachel resented being expected to help her mother, particularly as her mother was often cross and irritable. Rachel herself became touchy and sensitive with her friends, which was making her unpopular with the form. She was full of admiration for her father, though worried because her parents seemed to quarrel a lot.

She decided to sort the problem out for herself. She had a long chat with her father, who was able to explain that the parental arguments were not as serious as they sounded, simply part of the way marriage worked. She began to appreciate points about her mother: for example she began to talk about the clothes her mother made her, the fact that her mother was paying for her to go abroad. She showed more tolerance and understanding of her mother and she became more accepting of her female role.

Rachel was feeling much better. But it must have been too much of a strain for mother, who gave up the course the next term. 'Mother used to take it out on me, and I used to take it out on other people. Now we are all much happier.'

Jill (13)

'I get very involved emotionally with some boys, for example, when I was on holiday I went out with a 15-year-old boy who is much older than his age since his father died three years ago. I was very taken with him. When I went home he never wrote to me and ever since I have long depressed spells and get really fed up and miserable. My mother says I'll get over it, but with all her worries I have not told her how miserable I get.'

This illustrates a common dilemma: not that mum was not understanding but that she was too busy and worried with her own problems for her daughter to burden her further. Part of Jill wanted to be independent of her mother, of course. When she came to see me her depression about her boyfriend seemed to have completely lifted. What she needed to talk about was the family strains which were basically financial, to do with buying a new house. She took a pride in her parents' achievements but the move was making her feel insecure as well. She felt she did not want to add to her parents' strains but she *did* want to talk about it.

Elaine (15)

'My mother and stepfather entertain guests a lot. That leaves me, so every night I go in the back room and watch television. This is the drawback of moving at my age. I moved seven months ago and know no one at all where I am living. I go out three nights a week but to organizations where I used to live so it costs quite a lot of money to get there.'

Elaine had adapted well to growing up, with her church and youth club activities. But her mother's remarriage and the move to another district meant another period of adjustment. Elaine liked her stepfather particularly as he made her mother so much happier. But moving house at this stage is unsettling even with your own father. Elaine had to face the loss of her immediate friends and the loss of her mother's company all at once. Her mother had been widowed for the last six years; life had not been easy but the family had unity and a sense of purpose. Elaine felt lonely and slightly hurt at being excluded from her mother's new relationship, particularly as her mother was having so much gay social life. Again this is something many adolescents have to face, even with their own parents. But at least they are used to sharing.

After seeing the counsellor Elaine gained sufficient confidence to talk to her mother about her feelings. She decided to break with her old church and club and to join local ones. She began to build up her new life. Her mother, too, adjusted to her new married state and found more time for her family. Her stepfather insisted that Elaine have more pocket money and a dress allowance.

Carolyn (13)

'I have three younger sisters. I have a very strict father. He's the boss in everything. My family are very strict Catholics, that is why my dad won't let us have fireworks on Guy Fawkes night. I haven't any hobbies. I don't really do anything. I don't go out much at all.'

Carolyn was 13 when she wrote this. A year later her father was still being extremely strict and intolerant. By this time Carolyn could stand it no longer. She met a boy in the park, and they went out together for the afternoon. When evening came, she did not dare go home to face her father with the fact that she had been out with a boy, so she stayed out all night, huddled together with the boy on the stairs of a block of flats. The police picked her up next morning and examined her.

The only physical harm which befell her was the effect of cold and hunger. She was not a hard-bitten sexy delinquent doing this for kicks, but a rather shy and serious girl, who had responded to her father's extreme attitudes with extreme measures of her own. Fortunately her boyfriend was, like herself, not a sex addict but simply rather lonely.

She came to see me after the police incident. She had come for counselling in the third year to talk about her father's attitude, so our relationship was well founded. She had learnt her own lesson from the long, miserable, cold night vigil. But so had her father: he allowed her to go on seeing the boy, who became a regular visitor to Carolyn's house. The incident had achieved something, though I doubt whether Carolyn's objectives were as clearly worked out as this.

During counselling she expressed a great deal of anger towards her father for being too domineering and her mother for being too passive. Then it emerged gradually that her father was not at all well himself, had family worries back home in Ireland, whilst mother was also very tired and preoccupied with father's problems. She began to see the family situation in perspective. As her father had now given her permission to go out she realized it was up to her to take advantage of this. Half a term after the incident with the police, she gave up Colin, her boyfriend, who was beginning to bore her as well as restrict her activities with his evening visit. She went babysitting occasionally, to a youth club on other evenings, not in search of boyfriends but rather a more general widening of her experience. She stopped coming to see me at this stage.

A year later she turned up again. This time the problem was that her parents were thinking of going back to Ireland to live; this had the effect of making her want to leave school rather than do the CSE of which she was capable. Through telling me about it she began to realize what she was doing. She decided to stay on, whatever her parents did. That was the last I saw of her.

She had come to me because she felt I was the only person she could talk to freely. She had used me at a time of great need. It would have helped her more if she could have established closer communication with her parents. She said that they were unalterable and she was probably right. Through counselling and her own experience she had tried to make the best of a strained family situation.

Alison (13)

'I have not got any brothers and sisters. No pets. When I grow up I want to be a Repsenonist. My hobbies are collecting records, boys. I've no particular friends. I like everybody but everyone doesn't like me.'

Apart from a certain lack of ease with her contemporaries Alison's main and very real problem was the fact that her mother was in hospital, dying. Alison herself was worried and confused about what was happening particularly as she was not allowed to visit her mother. Father returned from his evening hospital visit exhausted, depressed and bad-tempered. Alison attempted to look after him but found him very uncommunicative. All this was of course very hard for her to bear. She really needed someone to talk to. I encouraged her to talk to her form tutor which she did to some extent, but rather self-consciously in the presence of other girls. Finally her mother died.

For a while her father became more possessive and difficult. He did not like her to go out because, he said, she was the only person he had left to depend on. She became moody, attention-seeking and difficult at school, and consequently even less popular with the other girls. She came to see me as often as possible for a friendly chat: to tell me her thoughts and plans in the way a girl might talk to her mother. After the first terrible shock both she and her father began to go out more and thus to feel less resentful towards each other. Once Alison felt more secure in her home situation she felt more secure with her friends and had less need to show off. She would probably have recovered without counselling but the counselling gave her a chance to grieve, to assuage her need to talk about her mixed feelings and get some of the individual attention that she now missed so much. I think this helped a lot.

Catherine (14)

Catherine's mother had left her and her father, who was out of work and under a psychiatrist. There were no nearby female relatives or friends to take on a supportive female role with Catherine. My role was just this: Catherine came for a friendly chat from time to time. Mostly she managed on her own; just occasionally her father's moods, unreasonableness and possessiveness got her down. As she grew up she was able to handle him herself with greater firmness.

Jane (15)

When Jane came in the third year groups it was clear that she had had an unsettling and difficult life but that she was making the best of it. When she was four her parents had separated and she had gone into a children's home. When she was eight she had gone to live with an aunt whom she loved and respected. However when Jane was 15 her mother remarried and took her back.

Jane was then faced with a real mother whom she hardly knew, a stepfather for whom she did not care and a little sister of eight whose existence came as a complete surprise to her. Not surprisingly she found great difficulty in accepting this new situation. Her work at school began to suffer and she became defiant. At the year mistress's suggestion she was glad to come for counselling. She was a girl of great spirit, courage and determination and all she needed to get back on course during this period of readjustment was a safe place to express her bewilderment, resentment and anger. She was confused by this sudden turn of events, resentful of not knowing what had happened to her mother in their years apart and angry with her sister who was a nuisance, stopped her getting on with her homework and had prior claim to mother's affection and attention. Her mother was stricter and less understanding than the aunt had been about such matters as going out. On one occasion, when Jane did not go straight home from school, her mother called the police and there was a big family row. After that Jane was able to go out more as she wished, and felt less resentful of her sister. For various reasons her mother became more critical of her stepfather and this made Jane feel closer to her mother, though it did not help the family situation as a whole. However Jane's school work remained uneven while she was still sensitive and vulnerable to the pressures within the family and too overwhelmed to take a stand for example about being given enough time and privacy to do her homework properly. Her own resilience and determination came to the rescue when she decided she wanted to work in a bank and realized that she needed good exam results to be accepted and to get the promotions she wanted. She worked with renewed vigour, achieved the necessary results and was accepted for the job. The motivation came from within her, which is why she was successful. But I am sure that expressing her mixed feelings about her family situation helped her to regain her sense of perspective. What she had to say was essentially personal and private to her family and it took time for her to work through her feelings. Thus the counsellor's role fitted her needs very well.

She did not dwell on her problems but used supportive counselling wholeheartedly until she felt strong enough to do without it.

COMMENT. In these examples it seems to me that I was a kind of supplementary mother-figure. Mother was too busy, too tired, too emotionally exhausted, too close to the girls or too distant, too active or too passive to fulfil their needs just then. My role varied of course according to the problem. But I was in the fortunate position of being able to give my full attention to the girl concerned without the constant interruptions which befall a busy mother. In the cases where there was no mother my role was even more vital. Non-possessive warmth, genuine concern and empathic understanding: this is what these girls needed and this is what I tried to provide.

Conclusion

Counselling is perhaps too grand a word to describe what happened in some of these cases. Applied commonsense based on respect for the individual concerned, perhaps even a simple practical suggestion, was often all that was needed. In other cases the counselling relationship, rather than anything that was said or done by the counsellor, was what helped these individuals face up to their problems. The girls worked out their own answers or took constructive action on their own behalf or decided to leave things as they were. They did not want anyone else to be brought into it. There is no real telling whether they were helped in the long term, or how long the effects of counselling lasted. Halmos says that counselling is an act of faith. It is one which I feel is worth making.

Chapter 8

Action

In this chapter I want to give examples of girls who *did* want other people to be involved in helping them to solve their problems. Sometimes an interview with the parents was all that was needed; sometimes a referral to social services or the child guidance clinic was the next step. I prefer for the moment to let the individual examples speak for themselves. It rapidly becomes clear that there is no set formula for getting a child the help she needs. To serve her clients to the best of her ability a counsellor has to learn to work in a flexible way. What works in one case may be completely inappropriate in the next.

Deidre (13)

Deidre was referred to me by her form tutor, who was very concerned about her uncontrollable emotional outbursts. Deidre was rather an aggressive tomboy. She had few friends in school; at home, she kept out of the house as much as possible, doing a paper round in the morning and going swimming at night. She was very independent, rarely admitting her emotional needs. She hardly ever talked about her parents; she certainly did not want *me* to see them.

I saw her once a fortnight for about two terms. She gradually peeled off layers of defensiveness like skins of an onion, until we reached her feelings. She began to talk a little about her family. She expressed her anger towards the school which she claimed had unjustly accused her of stealing. At this stage her form came for group discussions. This was useful to her for it gave her more confidence in me. I was pleased to find her quite well integrated in the group, despite her claim that she had no mates. Interestingly she did not swear at all in the groups though this was something staff frequently complained about. After the discussions I found her much less defensive.

Her relationship with her form tutor was the next problem to be faced. She was very antagonistic towards the tutor and provocative beyond the point of endurance. I was wondering what, if anything, to do about this when fortunately the form tutor came to discuss with me the angry feelings that Deidre provoked in her and the effects this relationship was having on the rest of the form. The tutor and the school seemed to be taking a lot of the anger which Deidre really felt about her mother and her home. Soon after, the tutor and Deidre had an argument in which they both aired their feelings. After that they felt much more kindly and positive about each other.

The next time Deidre came to see me she was a new girl. She thanked me for all I had done, something totally uncharacteristic of her 'old self'. She suddenly revealed a whole host of relations living near her whom she had never mentioned before. She had fallen in love, which helped her tremendously to admit her emotional needs! She decided to stay on and do a typing course instead of leaving early.

I saw her a little more, just in case this was a passing phase only. We had had stages before when she had become happier but it had never lasted. It was not until she had worked through her angry feelings that she could live more peaceably. She told her mother about her boyfriend which at last brought her closer to her mother. Her tutor reported that she settled down after that.

Marjorie (13)

Marjorie and her best friend came together because they said that everybody in the form laughed at them. They were rather sensitive girls—a ready target for the form's high spirits. Even their form tutor appeared to them to side with the rest of the form against them. There seemed to be only two ways out of this: to develop a thicker skin, or to talk it over with the form tutor and the form. They tried both. I did nothing except make myself available should they want to talk it over again.

Jessica (14)

Jessica said her form tutor was always picking on her. Very often this simply means that the girl concerned is insecure for some other reason, perhaps in her relationships at home. In this case there *seemed* to be no reason for Jessica to be extra sensitive. I felt sure that even if the form tutor *were* picking on her this was something unconscious or irrational. Jessica decided to make her feelings known to her tutor. Her tutor had not realized the effect she was having on Jessica. After that Jessica felt she was no longer victimized. I said nothing to the form tutor about the incident.

Annette (14)

Annette did not refer herself to me. A member of her form came on behalf of the others because the whole form was worried about her. She was large, rather pasty and lethargic. The girls in her form alleged that she smelt and was also a Lesbian. They deduced this from the fact that she often took girls' arms or put her hand round their waists. The form was beginning to find her unacceptable and wanted no more to do with her.

I said that there was nothing *I* could do as this girl had not come to me for help. As the girls in her form were worried about her, there was probably plenty *they* could do themselves to make Annette feel more lovable and acceptable. Was this Lesbianism or was it simply a great need for affection? Was there anything in her home situation which might account for her behaviour? What effect did it have on Annette for the form to reject her just now? Was the form tutor worried too? There were in fact many good reasons why Annette should have felt unhappy and starved of affection. The girls and their form tutor worked out their own practical solution. Annette did come to me in the end but already much helped by the support instead of the rejection of her form.

COMMENT. These girls' personal problems were affecting their relationships with the staff and pupils. I did not act as intermediary but left them to work out their difficulties for themselves. It was only when a member of staff approached me to discuss her side of the problem that I felt able to help without undermining her position or appearing to tell her what to do.

Susan (13)

'My name is Susan. I am 13. I have two sisters and one brother aged 14, 11 and 12. I live in a house.'

When I saw her in the group she was quiet and well behaved. A year later her mother came up to school to say that she was impossible at home. This surprised everyone because she had suddenly blossomed at school into a most responsible school citizen. When she came for counselling, her main feeling was that her two sisters were favoured, while she herself did a lot to help but was never appreciated by anybody. Her older sister was by now out at work, which meant that Susan had been ascribed the role of chief mother's help, formerly her sister's job. What is more her sister expected to be waited on when she returned from work, which enraged Susan's jealous feelings further. Although she was paid for her help Susan felt that no one appreciated her efforts (which indeed were probably loaded with resentment). She hardly ever went out. Home life became a grudging prison house; school was in the equally unreal state of seeing all the 'good' side of Susan's character.

Susan agreed that it might help for me to see her mother. Her mother, slightly suspicious of what I was up to and anxious to put her side of the case, was glad to come up to school.

Her mother talked a great deal. At the end of the interview she had begun to question her own attitudes. She was proud to find Susan so well regarded in school: this aroused a wave of positive feeling in her. She recognized that Susan might need to let off steam at home. She sympathized with Susan's position as the second of four because she remembered how she had felt in the same family position: jealous, overlooked, unappreciated. She thought of various activities Susan could take up to get her out of the house more. She decided to confide in her more.

The effect on Susan was that she began to communicate better with her mother; going out helped her to relax more and brood less. She began to make Christmas presents for her family: stuffed toys, clothes. These were warmly and fondly received. Her older sister sometimes set her hair and lent her clothes. Her mother took her out during the holidays and together they chose a dress.

If this had been a really deep and long-term problem of family relationships, one interview between the mother and myself would have had no effect. The problem was one of adjustment to a new stage of development and status within the family. The interview with the mother helped the family as a whole to pay more heed to Susan's needs, which helped Susan in turn to appreciate her home in more realistic terms.

Rose (15)

Rose was a West Indian. Her problem was basically that her mother was ambitious for her and worried that she might become pregnant which would stop her completing her education. As a result she never allowed Rose to go out, told her off if she ever saw her in the street with a boy and constantly checked the dates of her periods to make sure she was not pregnant.

Rose herself was an attractive and hard-working girl who, in the absence of any other outlet, began to fantasize about the only men in her life, her stepfather and the lodger. In the third year she had talked to me about the attraction she felt for her stepfather, though it seemed to be no more than a twinkle in her eye. She came back in the fourth year because, she said, the lodger had tried to make love to her. It was hard to assess what had actually happened, though intercourse did not take place. Rose had told her mother about it and was also willing for me to see her mother. This supported my view that she had provoked this dramatic crisis in order to bring home to her mother how desperate she felt about being cooped up all the time. She was also using me to help her make this point to her mother.

Rose's mother was concerned about her but she was more worried about her educational progress than about what had happened with the lodger. She wanted her daughter to complete her education and get a good job before getting married. She said that Jamaican boys were not trustworthy; this was why she did not let Rose out more. Her main complaint about her daughter was the total lack of communication at home: Rose did not tell her anything about what she was thinking or what she wanted to do when she left school.

Mother also needed practical help about Rose's future career. To this end I put her in touch with the form tutor and careers teacher. She left saying that it might help Rose to grow up more if she went out occasionally; she wouldn't mind if Rose went to a youth club or to evening classes, as long as she knew where Rose was. Rose herself was confused about her career: she needed the interview which we arranged with the careers officer.

Rose and her mother began to communicate better, by discussing her career and by talking a little more about boys in realistic terms. Rose was allowed to go out. She went on to be a nurse and as far as I know her mother's fears proved unfounded. But without counselling and help in communicating with her mother at a critical stage she might have been forced to more extreme measures.

Margaret (12)

Margaret was referred to me by her tutor in the second year because she was rather withdrawn and shy in school, yet her parents had complained that she wore make-up and was boy-mad. She certainly looked rather shy, frightened and tired and did not talk easily. Sometimes she would remain silent, sometimes she would talk, sometimes she would write me a story or draw.

She gave permission for me to see her mother early on. Her mother explained to me the significant fact that she herself was seriously depressed and had been receiving psychiatric treatment for some years. Margaret had expressed some of her anger towards her mother by putting on make-up and provoking a big row. More normally she cut herself off from the family when at home and escaped into a world of fantasy largely stimulated by her addiction to television. She had considerable creative ability which allowed her to express her feelings in her writings and drawings, in a rather macabre and powerful way.

I wondered at this stage whether Margaret herself needed psychiatric help; however one of her worst fears was of being like her mother, so she was completely against the idea and her parents only reluctantly for it. The interview with the mother had helped to clarify this for me, though I certainly also discussed the case with the educational psychologist.

Part of Margaret's problem was to *accept* her mother's condition instead of hiding from it. Another part of it was her own guilt in thinking it was her fault that her mother had repeated attacks: after her outburst with make-up, mother had become ill again; the same thing happened the next time Margaret had a row with her mother, except that this time mother went back into hospital for a while. When Margaret first came to see me she could not talk about her mother at all. When she spoke she would avert her gaze, never smile, as if this helped her to hide her guilty family secret. After I knew about her mother she was able to look at me directly.

When her mother went into hospital during the school holidays Margaret was able for the first time to take over the running of the house, with father's assistance. At last she could do something for her mother. This helped to assuage her guilty feelings and awakened pride and mutual respect between herself and her mother. Margaret found she could take on the feminine role without breaking down or becoming just like her mother. Indeed she became stronger and more positive through the experience. When her mother came out of hospital she and Margaret were able to communicate in a way which had hitherto been impossible, partly because previously Margaret was afraid to say much in case she triggered off another attack.

Because Margaret was more confident and less defensive her father was able to talk to her in an adult way about her mother's illness, which helped her to understand her mother better. In school her form tutor observed that she was still rather shy but that she did communicate well with her two best friends; she also laughed more and answered in class more.

COMMENT. In these cases I saw the mother once only. The interview served two purposes: it helped me in deciding whether a referral was necessary; it also increased the parents' awareness of their daughter's needs and possibly helped them to rethink their own attitudes. This is hard to judge: all we can say is that, as far as the girls were concerned, their problems worried them less from that point on.

Social services

Bridget (13)

'My Mother and Father are divorced. I don't see my Father much. I don't particularly want to, he's no good. We had a difficult time at first then my Mum met this man, Sid. He's nasty, not cruel or wicked, just deceitfully nasty. He nags a lot and watches me so that at the slightest fault he can call me selfish and lazy. Well, I'm not. Him and my Mum have terrible rows. I've witnessed some awful scenes. She's always telling me what she's done for me. I'm tired of it.'

At this stage Bridget was so tired of it that she wanted to leave home, be taken into care, anything. With Bridget's permission I consulted the social services, who also saw Bridget. There were no legal grounds for taking Bridget away from her mother and indeed it soon emerged that Bridget did not really want to leave her mother, only to escape from Sid, whose attempts to take on her father's role as disciplinarian thoroughly irked her. In consultation with the social services it was decided that as I had easy access to Bridget and more time than the social worker for preventive work, I should give Bridget the supportive counselling she needed to work through her problems.

I saw Bridget's mother early on; this helped a little in giving mother and daughter more awareness of each other's needs. I tried to get social casework help for the mother too but she resisted. In the end there was nothing to be done except for me to provide for Bridget a secure and steadfast adult relationship while she grew up and out of her difficulties. In school she was no cause for concern except for a general feeling that she could do better. Once she came to accept her difficult home situation and mature in spite of it her work began to improve too. 'I know it's up to me now and so there's some point in working.' Previously she had hidden behind her problems and taken no initiative in helping herself make the best of it.

Faith (15)

In the third year groups, Faith was ordinary, not precocious or conspicuous in any way, a Girl Guide and member of the St John's Ambulance Brigade. A year later she came back spontaneously. She looked completely different: eye make-up, modish hair style, fully developed figure. She had been going out with a boy with her parents' permission. He had recently gone to prison on a drugs charge. Her parents had suddenly clamped down completely on all out-of-home activities. Relationships between Faith and her parents had completely broken down. Father had sent for social services, threatening to get rid of her and put her in a home. There was no case for removal from home but father said she could set up on her own just as soon as she was legally old enough.

Unfortunately as part of her general rebellion Faith decided to leave school early, particularly as school too had had to punish her. I contacted social services who undertook to keep an eye on her and offered support to the family should they ever need it. What interested me in this case was the fact that Faith regarded social services as an arm of the law, brought in against her as a weapon on her parents' side. She kept from them her hurt feelings about being apparently rejected by her parents. Underneath her tough and defiant exterior she felt vulnerable and hurt. She found a job she wanted, as a punch-card operator, and she left.

Maria (15)

'I don't like being with a lot of people because I feel too shy. I prefer to be with one or two friends that I know. I find it a great problem because I am foreign and am a different colour from other people to mix with them. I find it hard to mix at home because I'm always being compared with my sisters at home and I am always in the wrong. I don't get on at home very well. My mother and I are always rowing and because our father does not live with us, I can never get a second opinion on any matter and many times I have wanted to leave home but never have. When I am old enough I think I would prefer to live in a flat with a friend or by myself. I lead a very jumbled-up life really which I have not yet sorted out.'

Maria's rebellion against her mother, her assertion of the contradictory aims of wanting to be independent and live alone, at the same time as feeling shy and in need of more support—all this is typical enough of her age group. But the extra complication of being coloured and having separated parents made Maria feel, at this stage, more than normally insecure and sensitive even though she usually cloaked this with an air of defiant confidence.

When she first came to see me Maria kept out of her mother's way as much as possible with the result that they hardly spoke. It seemed to me that mother was having to take all the blame for the colour problem (father was white) and also for the broken marriage.

Maria came to see me on and off for about a year during which time she gradually became more sympathetic towards her mother. There were many factors which helped this: she had gained in maturity; her father had come to live near her, which had given her an opportunity to test out what he was really like; she had come and talked to me about her feelings when she felt the need.

At the end of the next academic year she came back to say that she and her mother were terribly worried about the way her younger sister was behaving. She had re-identified with her mother to the extent not only of understanding her mother's problems but of sharing her worries, not just about the sister but also about health and finance. The mother telephoned me and I was able to put her in touch with the most appropriate welfare agency, in this case social services.

Christine (14)

Christine referred herself after the third year group discussions. It became clear from what she said that several welfare agencies were working with her family, which had many problems. Christine herself was the one member of the family dubbed sufficiently normal not to have a caseworker of her own at that time. She was obviously carrying and covering over a lot of strain and glad to come across someone in whom she could confide.

With her permission I got in touch with social services, who were the agency principally concerned with this family. It was important for me not to disturb this child by increasing her anxieties; it was also important for me to work with, not against, the other agencies involved, to minimize contradiction and duplication.

It seemed to me that my role was to keep our discussion to the normal, the positive and the good. If Christine should need to talk more deeply it seemed better for her to return to the therapist she had seen as a young girl. So for example I took care to praise Christine for the role she took within the family of supporting her mother physically and emotionally. My consultation with social services had served to clarify the limits of my role in relation to this particular child.

COMMENT. In these cases the counsellor worked with social services in various different ways. Each time it was important for the counsellor to consult social services as early as possible in order to work out their respective roles, which varied according to circumstances. In several instances not quoted social services referred to the counsellor for preventive supportive counselling girls whose problems were potentially serious but about which no legal action could be taken. The counsellor had easier access to these children and more time for this kind of preventive work, provided the girls themselves accepted the idea of counselling. If not there was nothing the counsellor could do to help.

Helping the parents

Irene (11)

In the first year Irene was often late or absent. Her mother wrote one day to say that the reason for this was that parental squabbles were making Irene ill. The staff referred the matter to me.

When I saw Irene she said that her parents were talking of separation. She often went to stay with her grandmother. Irene agreed that I should see her mother but the mother resisted this by saying that her husband had come back and everything was better. Later however the mother requested help from me and I made a home visit. Mother told me something of her troubles but it was clear to me that I could not take her on as a client and that one interview would make no impact on her many real problems. I suggested that the family welfare association might be able to help her. Mother phoned for an appointment and social casework began. After that I saw Irene only occasionally. In this case helping the mother was the key. Luckily the mother was prepared to accept help which is not always the case.

Monica (15)

Monica was in a form which happened to be predominantly bright and middle class. She herself was intelligent but from a completely different social background. She was the youngest daughter of a large family, with older brothers and sisters in their thirties. Her father was out of work and in fact had left home. When Monica came after the group discussions she told me of the family's circumstances but on no account wanted the school to know of the hard times facing her family.

At this stage she did not even receive free school dinners. I explained that these could be arranged and possibly a grant too, for clothing and maintenance. The school would naturally have to know that she was eligible for free dinners but the details of her family circumstances would be regarded as confidential if this was what she really wanted.

I wrote to the mother telling her where she could get help if she wanted it. The mother was extremely relieved and immediately went for help. Up to that point she had not known where to go and she had felt too ill, desperate and worried to find out.

The education welfare service which organized financial help on her behalf also arranged a case conference, during which it was decided that the mother would be helped by the family welfare association and I would continue to see Monica.

Unfortunately in this case social pressures were too great for Monica to get the education she deserved. Although her mother got a part-time job and some social security benefit through the help of the family welfare association, money was still short and Monica felt that she should be making a financial contribution instead of staying on at school. There was more to it than this. She already felt different from the other girls in her form; her progress had been impaired by various illnesses and absences and a general lack of motivation. Her mother wanted her to stay on to get qualifications but Monica did not like the thought of struggling on, studying every evening, having no clothes to go out in and no time for boys like all her mates.

The careers teacher arranged an interview with the careers officer; with Monica's permission I also sent in a report. She went to work in a computer firm. The family welfare association kept in touch with the mother.

COMMENT. Getting real help to the parents is sometimes difficult and often unacceptable to them. These are two examples where through the counsellor the parents themselves were put in touch with a casework agency and began to get to the root of their problems. The second example shows the importance of having a problem case discussion when more than one agency becomes involved. Our respective roles were defined to avoid undue overlap and duplication.

The family welfare association caseworker and I were able to work closely together which had advantages for our clients too.

Judy (13)

'My hobbies are reading and writing plays. I love visiting historical buildings. I loved school but now it is different as I seem to take things more seriously. I would like to be a history teacher. I would like to teach 11-year-olds who have to try hard to keep up with the rest of the class. The one setback is that I am not so good at written work so teaching is out of the question.'

She was an only child, serious, conscientious and somewhat anxious. Her desire to teach children with learning difficulties stemmed from her own experience at junior school where a particularly skilled teacher had inspired her confidence. Her work had been going quite well but suddenly it had got harder and she was having to face her limitations. To some extent her tenseness and moodiness seemed to be related to her monthly periods which had recently started. She was reassured to realize this. It was difficult to assess at this stage her ultimate academic level; she talked about this to her form tutor who was able to say that she might be capable of O levels, though not without a lot of determined work. In the meantime we discussed various alternative jobs which might fulfil her aim of helping others with learning difficulties, yet require fewer academic qualifications. I put her in touch with the careers teacher and the careers literature. She finally came to say she thought she worried too much about her work, which only made it worse. She had decided to concentrate on doing as well as possible but not to worry any more about which job she finally did because after all there were many ways of helping people.

COMMENT. I give this one example, though I can think of several others, of a careers problem which was really a personal problem. The careers teacher could have handled it from the start if it had reached her at this early stage. I was lucky in coming across Judy *before* her ambitions became too rigid and in having the time at my disposal to support Judy while she readjusted her sights.

Linda (13)

Many of the girls I see have problems which are not apparent in the classroom situation but this was not the case with Linda. From the moment she arrived at the school she was persistently aggressive, rude and violent. She hit other girls; she swore. The school attempted at the outset to refer her to the child guidance clinic but their every contact with the family was greeted with hostility.

When Linda met the counsellor in the third year discussions she decided she needed help. She wrote in her autobiographical note: 'Lots of children call me names, but it upsets me, and I squabble and fight them, then I lose my friends. I do not get on with teachers, I don't know why, but I don't.' The fact that she wanted to know why showed that there was some possibility of helping her. But the help had to be gentle and at Linda's pace; otherwise the opportunity of helping her would be lost. She resisted, as was hardly surprising, any suggestion that her parents should be brought in with a view to attempting yet again a psychiatric referral. She said they would be angry and refuse to co-operate. As this was borne out by the previous experience of the school it was accepted. But Linda herself could have some help from the counsellor and it was felt that some help was better than none. Many of the staff had tried at various stages to help Linda but she was particularly difficult to help in the authoritarian setting.

Linda used the counsellor very well at first, expressing considerable hostility and anger to the world in general and becoming as a result less aggressive in the classroom situation. But she did not come for counselling consistently; she used the counsellor as she wished, staying away for half a term, then coming back, spontaneously, when the situation got out of hand.

In the fourth year, she gained immensely in poise and maturity yet was still subject to outbursts beyond her control. Her parents began to express concern that her work was not going as well as they had hoped. This was the moment for the counsellor to press for psychiatric help. Linda herself now accepted the need for this and the parents realized that the school was genuinely concerned about Linda's welfare and that this was not a question of a passing phase in Linda or mismanagement on the part of the staff.

The counsellor's role had been to support Linda in so far as she was able and prepare her for specialist help when the time came. It is to be added that the staff generally were working to this end.

Joy (16)

In the third year groups, Joy had been quiet, sensible, without problems. In the fifth year she became aware that she was lacking in confidence in her relationships with other people, that she was frightened of boys and never mixed with them and that she was turning more and more to her studies to avoid facing her problems. She hardly ever went out, nor did she want to. It was not apparent that she felt like this; she was sensitive, industrious, perhaps a little shy. She kept her worries very much to herself.

In talking to the counsellor she began to reveal her fears and anxieties which appeared to go deep and to have origins in her infancy. She was pleased for the counsellor to see her mother; both accepted the counsellor's recommendation that it would be wise to ask for a diagnostic interview at the child guidance clinic. This meant that if necessary (as in fact it was) she could be helped by therapy to work through her difficulties at a stage when she was flexible and easier to help. This was indeed preventive rather than remedial work. Without the counselling service and the trust Joy showed in it it seems to me that Joy's problems might have gone unnoticed until they caused her to break down. This way she never reached breaking point. She went to the child guidance clinic for therapy for two years. I discovered later that she had then read sociology at university and herself became a social worker.

Mandy (14)

'I have a half-sister and half-brother, ages three and four years. My father lives quite near. I often go and see him. I miss him terribly. As he is engaged I hope he will soon get married so I could live with him. I have a stepfather and I don't like him as much as my real father but I suppose he's alright.'

She did go to live with her father. It did not work out and she was soon back with her mother. She came occasionally for counselling but only when she was fed up. She may have recognized that her life was basically insecure and that this fact was unalterable, but that it cheered her up to have an occasional chat. She was also ambivalent about me. On one occasion her mother had forbidden her to talk about family matters to me. Mother had later rescinded this but after that I felt Mandy was always slightly inhibited in what she said.

When it became clear that I was not going to be able to refer Mandy for psychiatric help (for she was extremely unsettled and insecure) because I had no powers to do this unless Mandy herself wished it, the school made more direct attempts to bring in help. A home visit was made by the education welfare officer to seek parental consent for a referral to the child guidance clinic.

This home visit illustrates vividly the difference between a parent's view of life and the way the child herself feels. The EWO concerned is not to be blamed for getting a completely different picture of the family from the school's. The EWO came back with reports of a splendid home, sensible mother, very concerned about the welfare of her child but sure that Mandy was just going through a passing phase. The school and I knew that the mother was defensive and did not really want to face the family's problems and that Mandy was insecure, emotional, unsettled and unable to work, living in a world of make-believe.

The breakthrough came in a strange way. Mandy stopped coming to see me. She went to live with an aunt for a while but that did not work either. Then one of her best friends was referred to the child guidance clinic. On the basis of her friend's recommendation,

Mandy decided this might help her. Her mother agreed; the referral went through. Mandy may have done this partly as a dramatic gesture but it does not really matter. We had all been working as a team to get Mandy the help she needed. The delay was of no importance for Mandy had not been mature enough to face her problems before. When she reached the clinic she was ready to be helped which made the clinic's task easier though by no means easy.

Diana (14)

'I do not get on with people very well. At weekends I usually watch television. I have only been abroad once but I did not like it. All the girls went with the boys and I just slept most of the time. I am not interested in sex or boys or fashion. I have always been fat or big built. I don't like cooking or needlework because I cannot do any of those things.'

Diana had worried the school for some time. Before she came for group discussion in the third year she had already been referred to the school doctor twice because the school was concerned about her size, her lethargy and her lack of friends. Diana had reacted in an extremely hostile way to the doctor, which meant that it was difficult for the doctor to help her. Diana was clearly defensive and sensitive about her problems at this stage.

When she reached the counsellor after the group discussions, she was ready to admit for the first time that she had serious problems: she had cut herself off almost completely from the society in which she lived and was beginning to wonder if life was worth living. She was seriously thinking of killing herself. With her agreement I saw her mother, who first took the view that this was a passing phase but who a week later agreed, as did her daughter, that Diana needed psychiatric help. A referral was made.

The counsellor was fortunate in coming across this case at a critical stage when there seemed a real danger that Diana might continue to resist the treatment she needed and break down completely. In this case the way we have structured our counselling service gave Diana the opportunity of revealing how she really felt. It was not obvious in school how near breakdown Diana was.

Vivienne (14)

In Vivienne's case it was the school doctor who was instrumental in getting her the psychiatric help she needed. Vivienne had been seeing me for two terms. She had a lot of deep problems, mostly to do with the emotional and financial insecurity of her background and her own inability to accept her female sexual role. She went around with gangs of boys who looked upon her as one of them. When she matured physically she was sometimes deeply hurt, sometimes very relieved to find that they did not recognize her femininity. She did not get on well with girls at school; she was often absent. Her one passion in life was horse riding.

She talked to me a great deal, hardly ever missing an appointment despite her general absenteeism. She resisted any suggestion of mine that she should go for child guidance or even that I should see her mother. Because of the permissive way in which we work there was nothing I could do to force this upon her. However the school was very concerned about her too; because she complained frequently of pains in the stomach she was given a special medical. The school doctor, in her more authoritarian position, was able to set a psychiatric referral in motion. In fact, Vivienne was well prepared for this by then and accepted the referral without difficulty. She continued to come to see me, which indicated there was something in our relationship which met her many needs.

COMMENT. These girls all reached the child guidance clinic eventually. Sometimes the counsellor was able to get them the help they needed quickly. Sometimes she was only able to support them until some other turn of events brought matters to a head. There is no one formula for making a referral.

These next examples illustrate non-action rather than action. This is something the counsellor has to face: for various reasons, she cannot always take action or continue counselling even when it seems appropriate. I have put these examples here to show that counselling is quite often a waiting game, hedged by frustrations and sometimes even blank walls.

Mavis (14)

'At school I am quite popular as I am a different person because I must not be selfish to the people around me in being moody, so I put on a happy face, but this is not me. As I say, I like to be alone, but this is difficult sometimes as people keep interrupting me, but I do need to be alone in a way I cannot explain. I cannot understand phonies who go around in a crowd just to be in. My mother asks me why I don't confide in her, but she thought I was being funny one time when I tried to explain myself so I never tried again. She is nice in her own way but she will never understand me. My father thinks that everyone should be happy at all times and if you are not smiling you are called miserable, but he doesn't seem to realize that he himself gets miserable sometimes but no one can say a word against him. Later on in my life I would like to live on my own.'

These comments sound typical enough of an articulate adolescent but in fact Mavis's sense of isolation and of being different was exceptional. She never quite succeeded in breaking through the communication barrier with her parents. She felt so different from her parents and her peers that she left school before she found her real self. She needed psychiatric help.

I tried very hard to get her parents' agreement for this, making several home visits. Mother eventually agreed but father remained adamantly opposed to the idea of her seeing a psychiatrist, which meant that her case could not be accepted by the local clinic. I continued to see her myself, taking care to discuss her case with the local child psychiatrist at intervals. Finally Mavis took an overdose of aspirins, fortunately without fatal effects. She told me about it the next day; together we told her mother, who upon my advice put the whole matter in the hands of the family doctor. He was fortunate in having a psychiatric social worker attached to his practice; she was able to continue to work with Mavis and keep a close watch on her after she left school. In fact leaving school seemed to help her to find herself.

I had been in a difficult position with this case, certainly carrying more than I was qualified to do and needing the case discussion which mercifully the clinic provided. Both the school doctor and I had advised the parents of the need for child guidance; when the parents refused, we could have left it at that. Yet at the time I felt some help was better than none.

Georgina (14)

'I'm 14 years old. In some ways I'm still rather tomboyish. I'm always laughing and talking. I love food and I'm always eating. I also love dreaming and imagine I'm in some kind of adventure. At the moment, I'm rather bored with life and would love to get involved in some kind of adventure.

'I'm an only child so I'm used to being on my own. I am very independent and could manage well on my own. I think this is because I've never got on with my parents. I look after myself really. My big problem is that I hate my father and have not spoken to him for a year. I don't like my mother much either. When I am old enough I have to leave home, but this does not bother me.'

She may well have approached me more in a spirit of adventure than in a quest for the truth, for although she talked a lot about her feelings for her parents she did not *really* want to alter the situation in any way. She was out every evening at the house of a friend whose parents she liked; in school she appeared cheerful and extrovert and, like many of her contemporaries, was crazy about pop groups. She had found an acceptable *modus vivendi*. She never told me what was at the root of her hatred for her father; she did not want to go into it any deeper (for example by being referred to the child guidance clinic), so we left it at that with an invitation for her to come back at any time. She had simply wanted to talk about what she normally kept to herself but for the time being that was all.

Jeannette (13)

All Jeannette wrote in her note was this: 'I have three brothers and two sisters. They are 14, 11, 10, 8 and 5. In my spare time I like to go swimming with my friends.'

This note is a clear statement at this stage that she did not want the counsellor to know anything about her. In fact she had serious problems in her relationships with her siblings. It is easy to interpret the note in retrospect. Anyone of 13 with so many brothers and sisters so close is likely to have problems. She doesn't mention her parents which is significant and her only positive statement is about her friends. She seems to be disassociating herself from her family and keeping herself very much to herself.

As it happens this was the case but the counsellor could not have assumed this from the note, indeed would not have presumed to assume this without further indications from the girl herself.

In fact Jeannette did not turn to the counsellor for help until about a term after writing this note. By then she was feeling totally alienated from home and school and talking to the counsellor was for her the first step towards restoring her relationships with her world. In fact such was her need to be independent of all adults that she chose not to come for any more counselling. In the end she got into serious trouble and was referred by social services to the child guidance clinic. In her case our permissive approach made it difficult to help her for she wanted help from no one. She provides an example of the limitations of the counsellor's role.

Stella (14)

'I do not talk to my father much as I am not over-fond of him and have lost my respect for him over the last few years because of family trouble. Through this a lot of my love goes to my grand-parents, though mostly to my mother.'

There was a genuine marital problem here which Stella kept very much to herself in school. The parents had been to the Marriage Guidance Council for counselling and the mother was also seen regularly by the family doctor for her nerves. I didn't see Stella many times for she seemed to have adjusted well to the family situation, to accept it, and to be unaffected by it. She did in fact show considerable dramatic talent, which helped her to remain confident and outgoing. The note itself shows dramatic flair though it is also surprisingly detached and matter of fact in tone. What was interesting about this case was that when Stella's parents began to get on a great deal better, Stella herself was very put out by having to share her mother with her father. She over-idealized her mother and normally made great allowances for her shortcomings. These became less tolerable to her when she had only a part-share of her mother's affection and when she was forced to admit that her father was not entirely 'bad'. She was beginning to see this when she stopped coming for counselling. It was too uncomfortable to face reality. In any case in all probability the basic marital situation would remain the same. Stella had already worked out a way of existing alongside it and it might only unsettle her to probe further at this stage. Self-insight is not always in the client's best interests; she wasn't ready for it then and so stopped coming.

Jonquil (14)

'I like my father and mother very much, but sometimes after I have been told off and shouted at, I think in my heart that I hate them, and when I'm old enough I would leave them and get a flat of my own. I don't always accept the fact that "tellings-off" are for my own good and sometimes think they *definitely* aren't. My parents sometimes cannot see why young people do wrong things, like taking drugs etc. They think it is their own silly fault for taking them at their age, but my parents do not realize it is the older people that started giving the drugs to young people and making money out of it.

'I don't rightly know what I want to be or do when I leave school. I think I would like to be a secretary or a punch operator as long as I could work in an office. If this were not possible I would like to work with small children as I like children.

'I don't go out a lot, but my sister does and brings her friends home and I am quite happy to listen and talk to them. My mother and father wonder why I don't go out and get boyfriends but I just like to stay indoors and watch the television and read girls' comics or books. I suppose really I will start to go out and about more when I really want to, but not yet and they find it difficult to understand. I suppose I find them difficult to understand sometimes, but we will all just have to put up with it.'

There is a negative tone underlying these wise but sad comments on the generation gap. Jonquil was not in fact as happy staying at home as she makes out here but the relatively unusual situation of having parents urging her to go out did not help her to summon the courage to venture forth. Her basic problem was insecurity about her parents' love so that their exhortations seemed to her in many ways a kind of rejection of her. She needed to feel much more confident about them before she was ready to leave them.

Her brother and sister on the other hand appeared to her to be the parental favourites. What is more she regarded them as attractive outgoing people, and considered herself shy and felt that her appearance was hampered by glasses. Another factor that contributed to her feeling of being different from her family was that she was intelligent, certainly A level standard, if not more, and was therefore able to argue with her parents with a degree of logic which made them feel insecure and resentful that she should win arguments. The other children were much more in their parents' mould, though Jonquil's relatively low job aspirations may well reflect a desire to remain acceptable to the family.

As far as Jonquil was concerned she found it very depressing to have her parents mock or block her every attempt to hold an intelligent adult conversation. She interpreted this as meaning that they did not accord any adult status to her, the recognition as a young adult which she needed to feel confident enough to go out.

We never worked right through this. Like many of my clients Jonquil only came three times. It is impossible to know whether she did in fact rethink her own attitudes to her family and realize her own strength sufficiently for her to become more tolerant and relaxed in her attitude to her parents. Three sessions might have done something with such a perceptive child. Perhaps not–her family relationship might have simply remained in her eyes an unsatisfactory one which in her own words she would just have to put up with until she was truly adult. I do know that her mother had in fact been suffering from nervous strain and when she went to the doctor about this and also changed to a part-time job, the atmosphere became more relaxed. I also know that Jonquil already had one sympathetic adult to talk to about her feelings, namely a young married woman for whom she baby-sat sometimes. So we did not prolong our counselling sessions.

If the clients seem happy to cease counselling for a while as Jonquil did, then we hope that they will come back later if the situation again becomes intolerable. But we do not *encourage* girls to have problems. If they appear to be coping reasonably well with their own problems without us, then we are able to concentrate more on the girls who really need our help.

COMMENT. These are all examples of cases where counselling had only a limited value. In some cases the individuals concerned did not really want help and within the permissive framework of our particular scheme the counsellor had no powers to see them unless they wanted to come. In other cases their problems were too deep or complex for the counsellor to handle alone, yet offers of more specialized help were refused. In cases of deadlock I always take care to ask the staff whether they are at all worried about the individual child. If they are, they are able to press for action in the ways they did before counsellors existed.

Conclusion

These last examples are for you to think about and discuss. They are typical of the sort of problem a counsellor may have to face–or a form teacher, for that matter.

Ann (14)

'Ever since I was nine I have lived with my great-aunt because my mother died and my father was separated from her when I was two. Because my Auntie is old (76) she don't understand or approve very much of the younger generation and when I wish to go to a quite normal place she will say no. When this situation arises I usually act deceitfully and go regardless of what she says, but I don't enjoy doing this for I would rather tell her. I am not allowed to have boyfriends but I do usually without her finding out and when I want any advice about them, instead of going to her I go and talk them over with an older woman I know. My Aunt expects me in at 9.30 every night of the week, but I never keep to these times. She never trusts me to go out and says before I leave that if I become pregnant I will go into a home. This proves that she don't really know what sort of a person I am.

'When I leave school I don't really know what I want to be, but I am going to carry my education a little further.

'I like to wear fashionable clothes and usually make my own, which works out much cheaper. Sometimes I see people along the street wearing way-out clothes, then when I have the time and the money I make something of what I have seen. I have many moods and sometimes I feel that I want to be noticed so I wear my way-out clothes but at other times I am shy and wear ordinary clothes.'

Gwen (14)

'I live with my nan and grandad, not with my mother and father. My mum left my dad when I was about two and my little brother was one. Because my dad could not look after us, my nan took us over. Then my dad went to live with another woman, taking my brother with him. He did not take me as my nan would be upset to lose both of us. They had another four children and come to live near us. Recently, my dad kicked my step mum out, so then, although I live with my nan, I looked after the children every night after school till he came home from work and of a Saturday. Then my dad and my nan had a row and I'm not allowed to go near my dad's house any more. It worries me to think of those children not being looked after properly. Nan is ever so nice, I like living with her but she's ever so strict and won't let me go out much of a night. She worries. It upsets me not to speak to dad but he doesn't want to know: I get really hurt when the other children aren't allowed to talk to me.

'I've gone all moody and even the girls at school have noticed how grumpy I am. I used to go out with boys quite a bit but I'm so fed up at the moment, what with nan worrying about me, and me worrying about my brothers and sisters, I don't seem to care any more.

'When I leave school, I don't know what I want to do, but it must not be a boring job. I would like to get married and have at least four children. I do not think it's a bad idea to get married young, but I don't think I will get married young. About 20-21 years old. I would like to have quite a bit of money to buy what I did not have, especially a good modern house. Although my house with my nan is very nice, my dad's house is not very nice.'

Wendy (13)

'I have two sisters and one brother. We all live in a flat. My dad has a bad temper but that's better than a clip round the earhole. My mum is a bit overworked and has just had a check-up at the hospital. When I leave school I want to be a nurse, then qualify to be a midwife. Can you help me about this? My brothers and sister sometimes drive me up the bend. What can I do about it? I love all dogs and cats, but the trouble is I have asthma, although it's going I hope. My mum at times gets me very angry and depressed.'

Lesley (14)

'Both my parents work. I have two older sisters. My mother is always going on at me, but doesn't at my sisters. My father is always telling me off for the slightest little thing. If I have a fight with my sisters I get blamed for it and called all sorts of names like slut etc. My sisters never get told off but I always do. My sister is nearly 18 and my Dad said going out once a week is too much of a girl her age. I'm not aloud to go out either. It's rotten. Just because I live an hour away from school, my parents won't trust me to go anywhere in case anything happens. They don't like my friends—they say they're not good enough and will only get me into trouble. I'm fed up with it. They never think about *me*. How can I learn to be grown-up?

Hetty (13)

'I have one brother of 14 and a sister who's 10. I get on well with my brother and not with my sister. I get on well with my dad who is strict but doesn't keep me chained up. I *hate* my mum and don't get on well with her. We don't talk and never want to. My sister gets me into trouble all the time (that's partly why my mother hates me). My dads away a lot on business. I miss him then. When he comes back, he and mum go out a lot, to parties and that. They often leave us alone in the evenings. The other night they got back before I did and there was a terrible row. They said I must have been having it off with a boy, but I never. They hit me and said I couldn't go out for a fortnight.'

Chapter 9

Outside bodies

Who are the people outside the school itself who are concerned with young people and who can help the counsellor further his objectives? How can the counsellor get their confidence and co-operation? Can the counsellor really do anything to help communications within and between the school, the home, the community and its resources? Should he attempt to do this or should he limit his role to work with individuals?

These questions are easier to ask than to answer; indeed there is no real answer, for so much depends upon the circumstances of each particular case. It does however seem to me that the counsellor who confines himself rigidly to the four walls of his counselling room is only doing part of his job. Counselling must remain the counsellor's main function; in the majority of cases it is neither appropriate nor necessary to bring in other people. When it is, the counsellor's skill lies in choosing the right moment for action, in knowing the different strengths and qualities of the local community resources and in having already established with them a working relationship based on mutual respect and personal contact. Like the relationship between the counsellor and the pupils or the counsellor and the staff, this relationship is not something which springs up overnight in response to the information that the counselling service exists. It grows gradually as a result of careful preparation and constant renewal.

Parents

Of all the counsellor's extramural relationships, the most important is with the parents. These are the people whose attitudes and attributes most influence his clients for better or for worse; it is part of his duty therefore to enlist the support and co-operation of the parents, if possible, and to work with them, not against them. Furthermore without the parents' agreement the counsellor is powerless to bring in the specialist help of experts when necessary. It is therefore essential that the parent/counsellor relationship should be well prepared and carefully handled. We have to remember that like teachers and unlike certain social workers the counsellor is in the delicate position of being able to ask children to talk about their private lives without parental knowledge. What are the parents' rights in this? What do they think of the idea of a counselling service? How much do they really know about it? Do they object to having their private lives and habits discussed with a stranger without the opportunity of putting their side of the case? What can the school and the counsellor do to reassure them, to help to perceive the counsellor not as a usurper of their rights and a meddler in other people's affairs but as someone whose work may ultimately benefit the family as a whole?

In our experience we have found very little parental opposition to our scheme. The head sees the parents collectively and individually before their children reach the school. She explains the way the school is run generally and tells the parents about the counselling scheme, stressing the fact that it is a confidential, voluntary and supplementary service. This is also explained in the school prospectus. To my knowledge no parent has ever objected or forbidden his child to go near a counsellor at this stage, though I suspect that this is partly because, with all the other facts that they have to absorb, the parents are far too stunned and overwhelmed to take it all in *and* react simultaneously. Neither have any parents, to my knowledge, asked for their daughter to be withdrawn from the third year group discussions.

When it has come to individual counselling, some half-dozen parents over the years have telephoned or written to say they object. One mother complained to the head that she did not like her daughter to talk about her marital problems, then proceeded to tell the head rather more than the child had told the counsellor. Other parents were invited to come and see the counsellor. As soon as they realized the way the counsellor worked and the vital fact that the counsellor kept confidential information confidential (a safeguard which does not automatically apply to what children tell their teachers) most parents felt greatly reassured and began to work *with* the counsellor. In one case a child was so inhibited with her counsellor because she had to report everything back to her mother that the counsellor gave up working with the child and took on the mother, whom she saw about once a term.

Something we have tried, and which we should probably try again, is to devote a whole parent teacher association meeting to counselling. This is how we spent the evening: after an introduction by the head, the counsellors each gave a short talk about their work and methods and answered questions. Then the parents were divided into small groups and given various problems to consider. They were asked first to discuss the situations, then say what they thought the parents should do. Most of the groups never got further than the first problem, which stimulated an amazing amount of controversy and disagreement. Here are a few of the examples:

Janice is 14. She has a boyfriend, Michael (16), whom her parents have met. She is allowed out with him until 9 pm. Last Saturday they went to a party and did not return until 10.30 pm.

Sally is a mature 15-year-old who goes round with some girls of 17 who are already working. Her friends invite her to come to a holiday camp with them for a week.

Julie is 15 and came home from her club one night looking very pale. She burst into tears and after much persuasion told her mother that a man had molested her on the common.

Sue and her parents have always wanted her to be a doctor. She is shattered one day to learn from her favourite mistress that she has no chance of achieving her ambition since her academic work is not good enough. She confides all this to her mother.

Maureen's parents had really wanted a boy first. Maureen herself (14) is rather a tomboy, always scrapping with her younger brother (10) whom her parents idolize. She resents helping her mother with the housework since her younger sister (eight) gets off scot free. She keeps out of the house as much as possible. As far as her parents are concerned she seems helpful and reliable enough when she is in. Her parents are very surprised to learn from the school that Maureen is restless and noisy in class, aggressive in the form and that she has been truanting.

The parents found it hard to agree (which is healthy enough) about what age a girl should be allowed out at all, let alone with a boy or older girls or alone. Some parents were relieved to find that when their daughter said 'but everybody else goes to parties except me' this was not exactly true. Other parents were left wondering whether they were not a little too strict—or too lax.

We hope they thought and talked afterwards both to each other and to their children about the difficulties of balancing their duty to protect their daughters against their daughters' need to grow gradually into independent and responsible young women.

Interviews with parents

In chapter 7 I gave examples in which it was not possible or advisable to see the parents. Although one of our general objectives is to improve communications between parents and their daughters it is often better for the girls to tackle this themselves without the intervention of a third party. In families where the atmosphere is already tense and explosive it seems unlikely that parents would give permission for their daughters to let off steam in confidence—yet this is what they need to do. In these cases asking the parents' permission for their daughter to be counselled might make matters worse within the family and deprive the girl concerned of the chance to express her feelings in a safe place. The counsellors feel no compunction about letting the girls talk without their parents' knowledge, because they know they keep the girls' confidences. So the counsellor leaves it to the individual child to tell her parents that she is seeing the counsellor.

In some cases I am sure the girls are right *not* to tell their parents. In others they judge astutely what is a good moment to explain, often using it as a way of introducing a discussion with their parents about their own problems. In other cases they tell their parents from the beginning: but these are the parents most able to tolerate the idea of not knowing everything about their daughters. After one girl told her parents she had confided that she was worried about their arguments they stopped arguing in front of her. I remember feeling that this was probably not the solution to their marital problems. But it would have been impertinent and out of place for me to have suggested marriage guidance counselling, particularly as it might not even have been necessary. Sometimes in an interview with the parents it is possible to suggest that they might be able to get help of this nature and to be more specific if they ask for details. But for the counsellor to tell the parents to go for marital counselling is rather like telling a teacher she needs a refresher course; it is not the counsellor's business unless her advice is specifically sought by the individuals concerned.

Sometimes a girl will ask the counsellor to see her parents. Sometimes the counsellor takes the initiative in making the suggestion. When the counsellor does decide that it would be helpful to see the parents she first gets the child's permission to do this. Some children are apprehensive about what may be said, particularly when what they have been telling the counsellor is a distortion of the truth. The child's trust in the counsellor may be shaken by a parental interview, even when the interview has been entirely as expected. If a child has been twisting the truth to get sympathy, the parental interview can help her to face what she has been doing. As long as the counsellor has not brought the parent in too soon, as long as the counsellor/client relationship is well established, this may be the turning point in the child's understanding the dynamics of her family situation. In one case for example Sylvia had given the impression that her mother (who was divorced) and her mother's boyfriend shared the same bedroom as herself. In fact the mother was very careful about where and when she made love and her boyfriend did not normally stay the night. What Sylvia was really trying to get across was the fact that her mother had not realized how sexually aware she was nor how much she needed mothering and guiding in her own sexual behaviour. I don't think this was clear until after the counsellor had seen the mother and the true picture had emerged. The interview with the mother helped Sylvia to communicate to her mother that she needed more of her attention.

The counsellor will see parents for a variety of reasons. Sometimes it is to help the counsellor assess the extent of the problem and decide whether a referral need be made; sometimes it is to get the parents' agreement for a referral to the child guidance clinic or the parents' permission for a discussion of the case with the child guidance staff to see whether they advise a referral. Sometimes the interview with the parents is enough in itself for it may increase their awareness of their daughter's feelings or help them to rethink their attitudes towards her. Sometimes the interview with the parents reveals problems in them so great that they themselves ask for help and can be referred to an appropriate agency.

What happens when the parents refuse to co-operate, particularly in giving permission for psychiatric diagnosis or treatment? If this kind of referral is indicated one of the counsellor's tasks is to reassure the parents that going to the child guidance clinic does not mean their child is a 'nut case'. She will show her own confidence in the clinic and describe in realistic terms what the parents may expect to happen if they agree to diagnosis. Even then parents often take a lot of convincing, sharing with a great many of our society the distorted and sceptical view that a psychiatrist is, as someone once put it, a 'cross between a witch doctor and a lavatory attendant'. The children themselves and the younger parents are less resistant to the idea of preventive psychiatric treatment, accepting that a psychiatric illness, like TB, is easier to cure in the early stages. The children who go for guidance have not usually reached the stage of being mentally sick. Even so it is sometimes hard to get across what it *is* all about: as one mother said to my colleague, 'She doesn't need to go to that clinic. She's not sick you know—it's all in her mind.'

It is not always necessary or helpful for the counsellor herself to see the parents. Sometimes it is better for the head or deputy head to do this, because the referral is being based on the way the girl has been behaving in school, which is something they know about and the counsellor has only heard about. With certain parents the authority of the head or deputy head adds weight to the recommendation, which makes the parents more likely to accept. Sometimes their authoritarian and judgemental role has the reverse effect—the parents are on the defensive and are not going to admit there is anything wrong with their daughter or the way they've brought her up; it must be the school's fault. 'She's no trouble at home, she never bleeding-well swears in front of us.' This kind of hostile parental reaction may come about when the head or deputy has not in fact been the least authoritarian or judgemental but when the parents have expected them to be so and have attacked even before battle has commenced.

With this sort of parent (and the school may well know from

previous encounters which parents these are) the counsellor can usefully present herself as someone outside the authority structure who is in no way criticizing or complaining about their daughter, simply as someone who is concerned about her general well-being and progress. If the reason for the child's disturbed behaviour in school lies in the family circumstances at home and this is something the counsellor already knows in confidence, then the parents are more likely to break down their defences and talk about the real problem, rather than cover it up; furthermore if they realize that the counsellor knows something of the truth they are less likely to gloss over their fundamental problem and slide away. But there is no guarantee of this either: why should parents tell the counsellor everything?

Take the case of Antonia: she appeared very disturbed yet the mother's account of the home situation gave no indication of why this should be. The counsellor said that she was nevertheless still very concerned about Antonia but that her mother was in a better position than she to know what it really was that was worrying her and how serious it was. The mother must have weighed this carefully: soon after she asked for a child guidance appointment. It transpired that the marriage was on the point of breaking up, something both mother and daughter had concealed in talking to the counsellor.

I know that many heads find themselves burdened with parents' problems: marital, financial, social and psychological. Yet there are again certain parents who never quite overcome the feeling of awe a head teacher inspired in them when they were young. This has nothing to do with the actual attributes of the head: she may be the most approachable of persons, yet some parents will only ever approach her wearing, metaphorically speaking, their best hat and putting on their best front. I have found this type of parent, once assured of the counsellor's trustworthiness, willing to confide some family secret which they would never on any account wish the school to know, yet which does have an important bearing on their daughter's problem.

In our experiment, when the counsellor first began to see the parents, the year mistresses or form tutors would naturally enough ask if they might also see the parent while she was in school, particularly if it was a parent who was hard to catch. We soon stopped this arrangement by mutual agreement. It was confusing for the parents and generally made them more defensive when they saw the counsellor, because in their minds she was mixed up with the 'powers that be'.

Yet even here we have learnt to be flexible according to the needs of the situation. For example in one case the counsellor saw the mother to express her general concern about her daughter and explain about the child guidance clinic; then the year mistress was invited to join the discussion to explain the exact way the daughter was behaving in school. The mother accepted the need for referral. This did not happen by chance: the year mistress and the counsellor had worked out their respective roles very carefully.

Home visits

Is school the best place for interviewing parents? Is it not better to see the parents at home because they are less likely to be defensive and hostile there? Is this not the only way to get hold of certain parents, namely the least co-operative ones, who have never been up to school even in response to a specific invitation? I know that these are controversial topics, which can be well argued on either side. My own view, based on my experience and a recognition that there are limits to the amount the counsellor can undertake, is that it is usually more helpful for the parents to come up to school to see the counsellor. Our normal procedure is therefore for the counsellor to write to the parents inviting them to come for an interview. She may follow the letter up with a phone call if possible to arrange the time and place. This will then be confirmed in writing. If it is absolutely impossible for either parent to come to school, even outside school hours, then the counsellor will arrange to make a home visit or she will ask the education welfare officer to make a visit on her behalf. Sometimes she will decide from the outset that it is better for the EWO to undertake all contact with parents. This point had to be carefully weighed every time.

The main reason the counsellors like the parents to come up to school to see them is that this helps them to conduct the interview in a professional manner. In the neutral setting of the counsellor's room, secure from interruption or diversion, it is easier for the counsellor to keep to her objective of helping her client, the child, by getting the parents' co-operation, and less tempting for her to fall into the trap of switching clients, of suddenly seeing so much of the mother's point of view that her relationship with her original client, the daughter, is impaired. Clearly part of one's professional skill lies in being able to face this dilemma and avoid being made to or appearing to align oneself either for or against the mother or child. But this may be easier on neutral ground.

Visiting the home not only risks impairing the counsellor's objectivity or neutrality. It also colours, possibly prejudices, her view of the family. Value judgements about the way a house is furnished or run reflect one's own experience and standards, more than they throw any true illumination upon the case in hand, but it is hard not to be influenced, inwardly at least, by what one sees. I remember once hearing a teacher's description of a home visit which brought this point home to me very well. The teacher was scandalized by the fact that at four o'clock in the afternoon the sitting room was untidy and dirty, covered with toys and washing. To me, as a mother, this did not seem to be an extraordinary or unexpected state of affairs; but this again was a personal judgement, not a professional one.

The teacher who visits a home and concludes from the fact that the house is well run, clean and tidy and that all is well with this family may be misled in another direction. Training for home visiting, whether undertaken by teacher or counsellor, is essential to avoid this obvious kind of pitfall. The essential question to ask is what will the visit do to help the pupil? If it causes the teacher to gossip in the staffroom or impairs the counsellor/client relationship it is not a constructive exercise. The home visitor needs to be aware of these dangers and to tread both carefully and purposefully.

Another factor which complicates a home visit and which may distract the counsellor from her main objective, is the number of interruptions a housewife may have in her natural habitat. The baby falls over, the cat spills the milk, the man comes to mend the washing machine, a neighbour calls to borrow some sugar. A housewife cannot say she is engaged and must not be disturbed for an hour. Coming up to school gives her as well as the counsellor a chance to concentrate in privacy upon her daughter's needs.

Another problem to be faced by the home visitor is being swept into some family drama and then being expected to pronounce judgement. The home visitor who arrives unheralded and unannounced is certainly asking for this kind of treatment. If the family are not in some measure prepared for the visit they are not to be blamed if they take advantage of the visitor. An appointment or at least prior warning of a visit is not only dictated by courtesy and respect; it also prepares the family so that they are not caught off-guard and the value of the interview diminished. But watching a verbal boxing match between sparring marital partners, and then being expected by them to referee and pass judgement and *withstanding* the pressures to become involved in this takes a lot of skill and a certain professional detachment. The counsellor in our definition cannot possibly take on the problems of the whole family singlehanded and at the same time serve the needs of the pupils in the school. If the counsellor does take on a lot of home visiting and work with families as a whole, then in my view she is not a counsellor but a school social worker, doing a valuable but different type of work.

What the counsellor providing a client-centred service for pupils really needs is a school social worker (or community family caseworker) to work with her. We may make here an analogy with the child guidance clinic staff: the psychiatrist works principally with the individual child, though he may see the parents in the diagnostic interview. The psychiatric social worker works principally with the parents. The psychiatrist and the psychiatric social worker work closely together, which avoids the situation of the parents or the children playing one social worker off against another. The nearest we have got to this situation is when parents have been going to the family welfare association for casework and we have been seeing the daughter; in these cases we have liaised and worked closely with the family welfare association with our clients' permission.

There is clearly a very good case for working with the family as a whole rather than with separate individuals within it. This is the trend in casework, based on economic arguments (no unnecessary duplication of social worker manhours) and commonsense (unity of casework purpose, balanced realistic view of the needs of the *whole* family). It can be valuable for a counsellor to arrange a confrontation between a girl and her parents, even between a girl, her parents and her teachers. But the purpose of this kind of exercise is to get to the root of the girl's problems in relation to her family and the school. It will not and cannot solve the family's problems though it may influence them. The choice for the counsellor is not between taking on a family's complex problems herself or doing nothing; the answer is to know where members of the family can get the help they need, always assuming they want to be helped in the first place. In the absence of a ready-made counsellor/school social worker structure, the counsellor has to be flexible and ingenious in thinking up alternative solutions, guided by the advice of professional colleagues. Sometimes the counsellor has to accept, whatever the dictates of his own desire to help people to be happier and more fulfilled, that not everybody shares his idea of happiness, or wants to be helped to change his life in any way.

Other agencies

When we began our experiment, our position in relation to the existing services for the welfare of children was ambiguous to say the least. Although our local education authority obviously knew we were there and why, had agreed to our appointment as an experiment and indeed paid us our salaries as off-quota teachers on a temporary terminal basis, our establishment as counsellors was not officially recognized. We were regarded as an experiment, but one for which the school rather than the local education authority was to take responsibility. There was no reason why any of the local community services for the welfare of children should take any notice of our existence at all let alone take referrals from us, make referrals back to us, engage in joint case discussion or work closely with us.

When we first began our work the head took care to introduce us to various key people in the children's services. It is fair to say that our relationships were not very fruitful at first, for reasons which are wholly understandable. For our part we were too busy trying to work out our relationship with the girls and the staff and to establish our identity within the school to have much time or energy for community work. For their part the social workers in the community bided their time, wisely waiting to see whether we were useful and remaining possibly somewhat ambivalent towards us. Why were we needed when their services existed? Did we really know what we were doing? Weren't we going to cause even more duplication and confusion than already existed in the social welfare services? Nobody actually confronted us with these questions. If they had they would have found us equally unsure about the validity of what we were doing. As in our relationship with the teachers, the onus of proof as to what a counsellor was lay with the counsellors. In a sense we needed to be left alone for a time while we worked out what we could do. Then when we felt stronger and a little more clear-headed we took the initiative in contacting the social welfare agencies again. We visited each agency in turn, feeling sufficiently confident by then to express some of our own doubts and being in a position to raise some practical problems requiring mutual co-operation. It was from this moment that our working relationship with the community services really began.

It seems incredible in retrospect that this obvious stage should have taken such a long time to reach. The climate of opinion towards counselling has altered so enormously since 1965 that it is hard now to remember what an effort it was then to define our role and demonstrate our usefulness to other interested bodies. Reaching the stage where we began to work together with other agencies was not simply an intellectual process. It took time. For us to visit each social welfare agency in turn, as we did, to provide in advance a written account of our scheme, to answer questions about it, to put questions of our own, to discuss an ongoing case where it was important to work together: this was a good beginning but only a beginning. One visit does not make a relationship but it is an essential first step towards building a relationship.

It is extraordinary how much *knowing* the people in a particular agency facilitates contacts with them. For example after we had visited each agency we would for a while find it much easier to pick up the phone and seek their advice on a particular legal point or their help on what procedure would best ensure a smooth referral if this was indicated. If we did not renew our contact at regular intervals, we would hesitate a little more to bother them and only ask for help in cases where we were *absolutely* sure we were not wasting their time. This is not healthy. It puts far too much responsibility for diagnosis and assessment on the counsellor and risks her sitting upon borderline problems until they are too far gone to be helped. In short it puts upon the counsellor the same limitation that teachers have when they do not have the opportunity to air their doubts in discussion.

So again as in our relationship with the staff it soon became clear that to be effective, community contacts had to be structured and they had to be structured on a regular basis. On the other hand there were so *many* social welfare agencies, statutory and voluntary, in the area that to keep up with them all would in fact involve the counsellors in an endless social work merry-go-round which would take them away from their clients and only be marginally useful to them. So we went for a deep relationship with a few agencies, confident that they would advise us who else to contact if necessary. Our work complements most of all the work of the education welfare officer, the social services and the child guidance units. It is with these three agencies that we have the most regular and constructive contact.

The education welfare service

Under our local authority we are lucky enough to have already an embryonic school social worker scheme. The existing organization has now been rationalized and professionalized even further. In its present form the scheme provides two invaluable services: it acts as a clearing-house for all social problems concerning schoolchildren, thus helping to avoid overlap and confusion; it provides home visitors, many of them voluntary workers guided and supervised by professional social workers. In the reorganized scheme the functions of the school inquiry (education welfare) officer and the voluntary worker are combined to make the school social worker (designated the education welfare officer). This worker is not expected to undertake intensive *family* casework, but to refer cases on to specialists where necessary. We find it a great relief to know that social work with schoolchildren is being co-ordinated and that help for the whole family is brought in where necessary. These are functions we cannot undertake, yet they are vital. We can co-ordinate the work within the school but it is not our job to co-ordinate work within the community.

Although we often see parents we have also found that in certain cases the welfare worker is better placed than we are for making a visit. The establishment of a friendly relationship between a family and a welfare worker enables the worker to keep an eye on the problems of the family as a whole so that when the time is ripe she may well be able to advise them on what to do. Sometimes this approach is useful for getting parental permission for a referral to the child guidance clinic though in an equal number of cases it is more appropriate for us to do this ourselves: it depends upon the nature of the case. It also depends upon the way the case has evolved. If the referral is entirely between client and counsellor it may be logical for the counsellor to interview the parent. If the parent cannot or will not come up to school, the education welfare officer may be able to visit. If the whole school is involved in the referral the staff may interview the parent on the grounds of the child's disturbed behaviour in school; or the school doctor may interview the parent on the strength of the child's strange symptoms, eg inexplicable pains in the stomach. Alternatively the EWO may be asked to make a home visit. The counsellor is sometimes hampered by the child's unwillingness to involve parents or accept the need for a referral. In these cases the school may take the initiative in making a referral, basing this decision on the evidence of their own ears and eyes, informing but not involving the counsellor. The home visit may well then be undertaken by the EWO; when the child reaches the child guidance clinic, the counsellor will send in her independent, confidential report (with her client's permission). This will be considered by the psychiatrist in conjunction with the standard school report, organized by the education welfare service.

When a family appears to have multiple problems the education welfare service will also organize a problem-case conference to which the counsellor can make a valuable contribution, provided again she has cleared this with her client. When a family's problems are severe enough to warrant a case conference, the client is usually glad for the counsellor to add her viewpoint to a conference which will take place in any case. At the conference are representatives of the education, school medical and education welfare services. If it does not seem appropriate for the counsellor to attend herself (for example if the head or deputy prefer to go) then her report can be considered by the conference.

Thus the counsellors are in almost weekly contact with the education welfare service. Sometimes we meet in school, sometimes we telephone, sometimes we write letters. The welfare workers are part-time: as we are, they are willing to be contacted in school by telephone, should it not prove possible to meet in school.

The social services

We are less closely involved with the social services, though we often seek their legal advice. We see them about once a term, sometimes less, but our relationship is sufficiently well established now for us not to hesitate to phone them. Whenever it seems that a case is potentially one which social services will have to take on eventually (eg care and protection, removal from home) we have developed the practice of seeking advice–either with our client's permission or without naming names–in the early stages. A social worker is then assigned to the case. He can be kept informed of the progress of the case and advise us on when or whether action is appropriate. Often there is nothing to be done, but by working closely with social services we ensure that we have not neglected or overlooked any way of helping this particular child. Unless action by social services is needed, this kind of preventive work is not reported officially to the school or education welfare service.

Cases of suspected cruelty or neglect, moral welfare and sexual danger put us in a difficult position legally. The advice of our education officer is that all such cases should be instantly reported to the education welfare service. Were we teachers we should not hesitate to do this. When teachers voice their suspicions to us we advise them to report the matter. When we are told about such instances by the children themselves we first make sure of the facts of the case, then discuss with the child whether it is in her best interests for something more to be done.

But it is not *always* in the child's best interests for something more to be done and often there is nothing more to be done. Our colleagues in social services may advise us that there is not a sufficiently strong case of neglect or moral danger for them to take action; our colleagues in the education welfare service may visit and tell us that all seemed well at home. Yet we may know that a child is unhappy or worried and all we can do is to support her until the danger is averted or the evidence is strong enough to bring in the law. Our first aim is obviously to prevent and avert a crisis. Our responsibility here, for good or for ill, is great and worrying at times. Yet for us to be simply secret agents of the welfare service or automatic referring and forwarding machines would not be in accordance with the principles of our particular counselling scheme.

Sometimes a social worker will phone us and ask us to take on an individual child for preventive and supportive work. This may be either because the social worker does not have time to do this himself or because the counsellor has easier access to the 'captive adolescent' who may also feel freer to speak outside the confines of the home.

If the counsellor already has a relationship with a particular child, referrals like this can work extremely well. On the other hand because coming for counselling is voluntary we cannot help unless we happen to have the confidence and respect of the child concerned. For example Sarah was in moral danger but not sufficient for a court action to be taken. The social worker responsible asked the counsellor to undertake preventive counselling with her. The counsellor had to make it quite clear that although she was aware of Sarah's problems and had tried to help her, she did not want help. The counsellor was out of touch with her; even if she had still had Sarah's confidence, she could not have guaranteed that Sarah would not henceforth get into trouble. Our method is permissive and entirely dependent on the co-operation of the client. Sarah did not accept the need for self-help. She needed firm guidance and strict control; the counsellor was not in a position to provide this secure framework. The person officially assigned to take responsibility for Sarah's general welfare was in fact a professional worker within the welfare service, known as the children's worker. She contacted the counsellor for a case discussion; the counsellor was able to put her in direct contact with the form tutor, who had already established with

Sarah exactly the kind of strict but friendly relationship she needed. The children's worker and the form tutor worked closely together. Sarah eventually reached the child guidance clinic.

In this case the counsellor had recognized and defined the limitations of her role. She still had a useful function in co-ordinating what was happening in school and putting the people who could most help Sarah in touch with each other. There is no reason why social workers or children's workers should not telephone school staff direct. Yet the counsellors find increasingly that they are telephoned by social workers from outside the school and asked either to take on a case or to help in some way. The counsellor acts as a useful link-man and sieve.

This co-ordinating and communicating role can often save time both for the staff and for the social workers. The social workers know that the counsellor understands and shares their ethic, whereas they may not be sure about the teaching staff unless they know them personally. The differences between the professional ethics of the teaching and the social worker professions may not be as great as many social workers imagine, but they must be recognized nevertheless.

Our work with social services is two-way: we benefit from their specialized knowledge, their experience and sometimes their unofficial casework supervision; we help them sometimes by taking on individuals for preventive work, sometimes by putting them in touch with the member of staff who can most help, sometimes by telling parents about their service so that parents may refer themselves for advice, sometimes by discussing with them a particular child in order to define our respective roles clearly.

Child guidance

School counselling is by nature most closely allied to the work of the school psychological services. It is with this service that we work the most closely and to which we make most of our referrals. In order to ensure that referrals are made which are both appropriate and timely we have established a system of regular case discussion with the two clinics that serve our area. One of the greatest difficulties for counsellors in an unofficial unstructured experiment is getting their work supervised to make sure that they do not keep cases beyond their capabilities, or perpetuate their own errors of approach. We have been extremely lucky in getting constructive help and guidance from our clinics, in particular from the educational psychologists. We have case discussion with one or the other every three weeks; we can also telephone at any time with complete assurance. Sometimes we go into the guidance units in which case the psychiatric social worker may join us; sometimes we meet in school. Apart from this the psychiatrist may convene a special case discussion for a new case, a joint case or a psychiatric case which the counsellor is having to keep because of lack of parental co-operation.

Diagnosis

In the general case discussion with the educational psychologist we raise first all the borderline cases where we are not sure whether child guidance treatment is appropriate, and then cases which are undoubtedly counselling cases, but about which we feel unsure, worried or dissatisfied ourselves. The educational psychologist will do testing for us if it seems appropriate, which is not often; usually she simply passes on the benefit of her much wider experience. When there is any doubt about whether a child needs treatment we ask the psychiatrist for a diagnostic interview: this after all is what he is qualified to do, and what we are *not* qualified to do. The counsellor is neither trained nor paid to take the kind of responsibility a psychiatrist will take for recognizing a psychotic or carrying a potential suicide. A wise counsellor takes medical cover in good time, recognizing (with some sense of relief) that it is not her job for example to decide what to do about a suicide threat and that this must be put in a doctor's hands, even if initially this has to be the family doctor rather than a child psychiatrist.

There is no doubt that the question of deciding what is normal and what is abnormal for a child of a certain age is very difficult. I am sure that if teachers took any definition of disturbed or maladjusted children literally, they would refer a large proportion of their pupils. (See for example the definitions given in the Underwood Report.[1])

The problem is in defining the degree of maladjustment, granted that many children show certain symptoms of disturbance at certain stages in their development. The Underwood Report says that 'a child may be regarded as maladjusted who is developing in ways that have a bad effect on himself or his teachers and cannot without help be remedied by his parents, teachers, and other adults in ordinary contact with him.' The symptoms do not in themselves indicate maladjustment. 'It is only when they are excessive or abnormal, when they prevent a child from living a normal life that investigation is needed.'

Defining what is excessive and abnormal is what is difficult, especially when we consider that there are bound to be a number of somewhat maladjusted children in any normal school, particularly since there are not enough special schools to deal with all such children, and that current policy is towards home based community care wherever possible. Both the Underwood Report and the DES Report on the education of maladjusted children make sensitive and illuminating reading for any teacher but, rightly, they do not provide a rigid yardstick for labelling children maladjusted.[2]

The counsellor has to have the same flexible approach. Rather like a good general practitioner he may through his experience of a sample of the raw population come to recognize which cases may need specialist help and which are within his sphere. But he does not do this alone; he recognizes that he is neither omniscient nor omnipotent. He asks the opinion of the form tutor and the advice of the educational psychologist and thus avoids either sitting on cases which ought to be referred or passing on every case which is in the least disturbing. In our scheme, the educational psychologists help to ensure that we make sensible referrals. When educational psychologists are so highly trained and in such short supply[3] this seems to me to be an effective and efficient way of using their expertise.

Referrals

When the counsellor does make a referral to the child guidance clinic she naturally first has to get the consent and the co-operation of the child and her parents; next she informs the head and the education welfare service, so that they may collect a school report plus any other facts already known about this child's background; she then writes her own confidential report to the psychiatrist and awaits an appointment. In the meantime she continues to see the child. After the diagnostic interview the psychiatrist will write to the counsellor (among others) to give his considered opinion and advice on treatment. He may convene a special case discussion to which the counsellor will be invited and at which it will be decided whether the counsellor should go on seeing the girl as well as or instead of the psychiatrist or therapist. Either way the counsellor will keep in close touch with the psychiatric social worker and with the child's form tutor so that two-way feedback (on how the girl is behaving in school and how she is responding to treatment) will be maintained. Occasionally when a child is being particularly disruptive in class the psychiatrist will come into school with his whole team of workers in order to hear at first hand what the staff feel about this particular child. This not only helps the psychiatrist in his understanding of the child's behaviour, but has the very valuable side effect of improving the relationship between the clinic and the school.

It is important to note that this simple mechanism for counsellor referrals took some time to establish. The counsellors could not make referrals at first because their position was not recognized. In the beginning we had three alternatives: to ask the welfare service to investigate and refer, or to ask the educational psychologist to refer, or to get the parents to refer themselves directly to the clinic. All these methods were cumbersome and long-winded. If we had already seen the parents, a home visit by the education welfare officer duplicated our efforts and caused unnecessary delay (to be added to the inevitable clinic waiting list, usually not more than six weeks in our case, but long enough). The educational psychologist was reluctant to duplicate the interview with child and parent, regarding this as an unnecessary extra spoke in the wheel and parents, however worried, were occasionally intimidated by the mechanics of making an appointment, apart from the fact that where possible the clinics prefer a school based orderly referral. The net result was to inhibit and delay referrals unnecessarily.

We finally established with the welfare service the principle that the counsellor would make clinic referrals direct, provided she also informed the welfare service so that it could retain its co-ordinating function. The child guidance units would not of course accept referrals from counsellors unless they recognized their existence and their value. Certainly their acceptance of us has helped us enormously to grow instead of wither, to learn instead of stagnate. We find it both encouraging and reassuring that the clinics will take some note of what we say: for example we may be asked whether we think a case is urgent. If we say it is urgent then the growing waiting list may be waived. Clearly this is something we cannot afford to abuse or misjudge but it results in the kind of *flexible* arrangement which should exist between a school and a clinic. More than anything else the idea of a rigid inflexible waiting list stops schools from using the child guidance clinic. If the problem is urgent, staff may feel that in six months' time it will be too late to help the child at all. In our area the waiting list no longer acts as an impasse between the school and the clinic. We have a hot line to the clinic which overcomes this obstacle.

The counsellor as go-between

I have already mentioned the important role the counsellor has in explaining to parents what child guidance is all about. The counsellor has an equally important role *vis-à-vis* the staff. Parents are not the only people to feel ambivalent about psychiatrists. Teachers too are often wary or sceptical of them. This attitude has been described as the 'magic wand syndrome': the teacher keeps a difficult child until he becomes absolutely impossible, then refers him as a last desperate measure. The psychiatrist is expected to wave a magic wand and 'cure' the child in a matter of months. If the child remains as difficult as ever, this is taken as proof that child guidance is ineffectual.

On the other hand child guidance units sometimes suffer from the 'closed shop' syndrome. So anxious are they to retain confidentiality and divorce themselves from the authority setting of the school that they omit to feed back to the teachers any comments or guidance. Teachers whose pupils have gone for guidance often feel insecure about how to handle these pupils in future. Should they be punished or will this make them worse? Should teachers turn a blind eye? What should they do if a child has a tantrum? It is usually neither desirable nor possible for the clinic to provide a straightforward answer. Clinic staff may modestly feel that they should not interfere with a teacher's professional techniques. In my view what the teacher is after is not a blueprint for helping Johnny but just some communication back to help increase her own insight. The counsellor can help both the school and the child guidance staff in this.

Without the support and unofficial casework supervision of the child guidance staff there is no doubt that the counsellors would be dangerously limited in their usefulness. As it is they have the reassurance of being able to share the burden of their responsibility, while in their turn they do much to communicate to the girls, the parents and the school what child guidance clinics are about.

The careers service

Of the remaining community services for the adolescent, the most important is the careers service. We know our careers officers and we do not hesitate to contact them if our clients feel this would help them. At the careers interview a girl might for example have been too shy to express her real needs; she might have been intimidated by the presence of her mother; she might have felt unable to explain her difficult home situation, which might be the key to a rather unsuitable choice of job. If the girl feels after the interview that for some reason or another she did not get across to the careers officer what she really wanted to say, she may ask us to arrange a further interview or help explain her problem. But this does not happen often because most of our work is with the third year children; we are not concerned with careers, except indirectly. We have relatively few fifth year girls on our books, and they more logically turn to the careers teacher at this stage if they are dissatisfied with their job choice. We have experimentally run group discussions for early leavers during the few weeks before they leave school but these have not been to do with job choice, which has already been made. Instead these discussions are concerned with helping to bridge the emotional and social gap between school and work.

The help we do give the careers officers is indirect, early and probably unknown to them. We always ask the third years in the group discussions what they want to do when they leave. This comes at about the same time as the first of the careers officers' talks to the girls, and also the third year choice of subject. In the groups we try to get the girls to think a little about what sort of people they are but we do not administer a self-searching questionnaire such as is used by many careers officers/teachers. We have not taken responsibility for this important task for the reasons I gave in chapter 4. But what we do pick up among all the third year 'don't knows' is a certain proportion either of unsuitable job choices, or of job choices dictated through social pressures rather than by any consideration of the girl's qualities and qualifications.

We have already considered the girl who wanted to teach children with learning difficulties although she was unlikely to achieve college entrance requirements. There are many other such examples: *Hyacinth*, who is a West Indian, wants to be a ballet dancer, though at 14 she has not yet begun lessons. *Aminu* from Pakistan wants to be a doctor even though she has been put in a non O level form. Helping these individuals to face their limitations without losing self-confidence or becoming defensive, so that they may begin to think realistically about alternatives, is a skilled counselling task and takes time. If together with the form tutor we can help a child work through these difficulties and face the moment of truth well before the careers interview, then we have facilitated the work of the careers service.

We can also sometimes help when there are emotional or social problems stemming from the home situation. *Dorothy* is capable of O level but her father has just deserted her and her mother, leaving them virtually destitute. She wants to leave early to earn money. *Alice* is very bright but from a working-class home, which sees no virtue in staying on. Instead of doing her homework she reads extensively but without purpose. If she is leaving at Easter, why work for GCE? *Helena*, a Cypriot, wants to do A levels but her parents insist that she leave early to help in their shop. *Carol* on the other hand shares her parents' negative attitudes towards education. Her only ambition is to marry as young as possible. *Colette* is leaving school early to spite her parents whom she detests.

Children with this sort of problem need much more than information about job qualifications and much more than exhortations to do better if they are to begin to do themselves justice. They may be helped by individual personal counselling to make a more rational decision about their future, though sometimes the social pressures of their backgrounds make it impossible for them to fulfil their academic potential. If the counsellor can work on the irrational and emotional factors involved in vocational choice early enough, this may again save the careers officer from the unsatisfactory process of eleventh-hour crisis vocational guidance. But the counsellor's influence in this sphere will be minimal unless the policy of the school as a whole is directed not just towards careers information and job selection but includes experience throughout the curriculum and throughout the school career of self-analysis and decision-making, with more consideration of how to motivate the individual child. Schools should heed also the parents who, if they lack aspirations for their child, may be the most obstinate and influential blockage to their child's progress.

Other community services

Our relationships with other agencies which serve children's needs are more superficial, but nevertheless well founded. We have met and worked with our education welfare officer. We know the local youth officer who has taken us round clubs in the area and who often helps to find a suitable club for a girl who says there is nowhere to go in the evenings. We know some unattached youth workers who are a useful potential source of help for the boyfriends of our girls. We know the Diocesan moral welfare worker who takes responsibility for unmarried mothers. We have met the probation officers but as we do not work with girls on probation overlap is minimal though could be greater. We use the family welfare association wherever possible for casework with parents. We have contact with several general practitioners in the area and also with the mental health workers who have been attached, also experimentally, to local group practices to provide an on-the-spot casework service for the doctors' patients. We have met the doctors who provide a counselling and contraceptive service in a nearby hospital. We know the local branch of the Marriage Guidance Council and the way it operates. This kind of knowledge and contact, built up slowly over the years, helps us to provide a better service for our clients, not because we actually use these agencies very often but because we know about them, and could use them if appropriate. Furthermore we find that as our service becomes known to workers within the community, they may take the initiative in contacting us, with the result that we are able to work together and reduce overlap and duplication.

The head, the counsellor and the community

In many schools the head or deputy takes on the role of co-ordinator of work with the social welfare services. This is an important job. Well done it may take up an undue proportion of a head's time. Inadequately done it may, through omission, fail to bring in help at the right time, which may indirectly hinder a child's progress. It seems to me that whilst retaining his power and responsibility as general overseer of what is happening in a school, a head could usefully delegate some of the daily tasks of contacting the welfare services to the counsellor. The counsellor for his part must be trusted to keep the head informed of important developments but not bother him with detailed accounts of every phone call.

Similarly the head who finds himself burdened with large numbers of social problems brought to him by parents may be tempted to take them on for himself at the expense of his other duties, or he may fail to bring in the service which exists to help just this situation. A head with a counsellor on his staff could save himself a lot of time and worry by giving the counsellor the time-consuming task of contacting the appropriate agency and arranging the first interview.

These communicating, co-ordinating and contacting functions of the counsellor are not of course counselling, but they are functions which could be aptly assigned to the counsellor, provided they in turn do not take up so much of his time that his work with individuals suffers.

Another role the counsellor may usefully fulfil within the staffroom is to keep the staff as a whole well informed about local welfare resources. To this end we have discussed the idea of a 'teach-in' for our staff, possibly combined with staff of other schools, at which representatives of the various social welfare services would define and explain their different roles and answer questions.

Ideally the counsellor in the staffroom should be available and able to give information to any member of staff on any incipient social welfare problem. If he does not know the answer he should know where to find it and have the time to follow it up. This at least is what we try to do. The staff consult us more and more about social problems, and we become gradually better equipped to help them. The staff seem to me to know more now about the social welfare services for children than when we began, to understand their methods better and to be more sympathetic towards them.

COMMENT. In working with parents and social workers as well as with staff and pupils, the counsellor has many different roles. Sometimes he is a communicator, sometimes an activating agent, sometimes a go-between, sometimes a public relations agent, sometimes a co-ordinator, sometimes a consultant. The counsellor has to learn to be flexible, to develop a good sense of timing, to wear two hats without becoming two-faced. Above all the counsellor has to remain genuine and loyal towards his client and to remember that, in many cases, involving other people may not only be unnecessary but also positively unhelpful or even harmful to his clients' best interests.

In most cases the counselling relationship is all the pupils want and all they need.

References

1. *Report of the Committee on Maladjusted Children* the Underwood Report (HMSO 1956)
2. *The Education of Maladjusted Children* Department of Education and Science pamphlet no 47 (HMSO 1965)
3. *Psychologists in Education Services* the Summerfield Report (HMSO 1968)

Chapter 10

The counsellor's problems

It is easy to look only at the positive side of what may be achieved by counselling. What about the negative side? What are the *dangers* of introducing counselling into our schools? How can we safeguard counselling standards? How can we evaluate the usefulness of counselling? How can we select and train the people most suitable to be counsellors? How can we do this economically? Are we sure counselling is the most practicable answer to the children's problems? Are there no alternative ways of achieving the same objectives? Should we do similar work in primary schools? Is counselling a priority when set against other educational/social problems? Can we afford counselling? Can we afford not to counsel?

I certainly do not know the answers to these questions; all I do know is that we must beware of introducing counselling into our schools without having weighed these points very carefully. There are many pitfalls and dangers in counselling. This is something that counselling enthusiasts, like myself, sometimes forget. Counselling may or may not be what the adolescent needs. A lot depends on the choice of the counsellor and the way the counsellor is trained and used. Even then the counsellor is bound to make mistakes: we must not expect our counsellors to be perfect. In this chapter I want to discuss some of the ways counsellors might be helped to do their difficult job, and also ways in which they might be trained more economically.

The limitations of our experiment

There are many deficiencies and omissions in the counselling system we have established; some we can see only too clearly; others have not yet dawned upon us. The limitations divide into two categories—first the human and personal, second the practical. In other words we make some mistakes because we are human and fallible. We have had to create and define as well as learn and grow, and this has added to the difficulties of the job.

On the practical side, there is no doubt that many of our problems stem from the fact that we are only part-time. For the time being we therefore have to leave undone many of the things we would like to have done. For example we would like to do more group work with parents, more group work and follow-up work with leavers, more group discussions with sixth-formers; we would like to begin our work in the first year and to develop more sophisticated and accurate screening techniques; we would like to follow up lapsed cases more systematically; we would like time to work more closely with the careers officers; we would like to set up regular discussion groups among the staff. All we have time for is to see the girls whose problems are so urgent and pressing that they want to see us sufficiently to take the initiative in seeking us out. We rarely have time for 'check-ups' and none for girls who can be equally well helped by others.

The result of this shortage of time is to put great pressure on us during the days we are in school. We spend most of these days seeing girls, usually for sessions of one lesson (35 minutes), occasionally for a double lesson. The quality of our work would probably improve if we saw individuals (or groups) for no more than half the day and spent the rest of the day talking to teachers, contacting welfare agencies, keeping our records and digesting what has happened. We do all our note taking, record-keeping, telephoning and letter writing from home which means there is no timetable limit on it. But I am sure that efficient administration is no substitute for being on the spot.

If we were to administer as well as counsel from school, we should of course need our own room with its own telephone. It is important for counsellors to be able to make and receive telephone calls in privacy, without being overheard by other members of staff. We should also need secretarial facilities: handwritten letters and reports risk not only being difficult to read but also looking decidedly amateurish. This raises the question of whether the general secretarial staff should be used by the counsellor for typing out condifential reports. My own view is that in a large comprehensive school with a fully developed guidance team, there would be enough work to occupy at least a part-time secretary (an interesting post for a married woman), who could be used solely by the guidance unit. This may sound unnecessary, but I cannot see otherwise how the counsellor can share with the head's secretarial staff what he is not able to share with the head. It contradicts the principle of confidentiality and privacy.

Teamwork in guidance

Perhaps we should consider at this point what I mean by a fully developed guidance team. It seems to me that in a school as large as ours there is ample work for one full-time counsellor of the type I have described, particularly if the important role of developing the staff's natural talents for counselling is pursued more thoroughly. To take on further functions might adversely affect the quality of the personal counselling which goes on. Yet we do no vocational counselling and no testing. Alongside the personal counsellor there is still room and need for a vocational or occupational counsellor, who might be a teacher released from teaching duties and specifically trained or a careers officer redeployed. In some areas already careers officers spend one or two days a week regularly working inside a school. An extension of this idea would give greater reality to the concept of teamwork in guidance, which is practically impossible without physical proximity, parallel hours and regular discussion. The occupational counsellor might undertake if desired the role of psychometrist (psychological testing); if the school wanted a lot of testing done this could be a job for yet another member of the team; alternatively there could be some interchange of roles between the various members of the guidance team.

This separating out of guidance into vocational guidance, personal counselling and psychological testing is recognized as being unrealistic. The division is made not because pupil problems, like Gaul, divide neatly into three parts, but because this simple division of labour seems more likely to promote efficient and effective guidance. The counsellor who sets no limits on his role may end by doing everything inadequately. He may be tempted to take refuge from the conflicts he has brought upon himself by escaping into the role of organization man, or by becoming too preoccupied with ranking and filing. Teamwork in guidance is not an extravagance but rather a way of ensuring that the initial investment in teacher-capital is not lost through insufficient backing. A new piece of equipment may cause more problems than it solves if the rest of the system is not modernized to fit in with it. There is always the risk with a new machine that it may be over-used and overstrained and so break down. We must also recognize that a new piece of machinery in itself achieves nothing; what is important is the *way* it is used.

In counselling the personal character and calibre of the counsellor is of the utmost importance. Whilst this is true of heads it is also true that their responsibility is matched by their accountability. The counsellor at his present stage of development is not really accountable to anyone. This is a dangerous state of affairs; an unfortunate choice of counsellor can have devastating repercussions for the individual and for the school, particularly as the bad side effects may not become apparent at first. This is a point which is often overlooked in British counselling literature.

Who shall counsel the counsellor?

However good a head is at judging the quality of his counsellor's work, seeing that his time is well spent, assessing what he hears about the way he relates to pupils, staff and parents, the head is not able to supervise the counsellor's work in any depth. This is partly because he is unlikely to be trained himself for this specialist role, partly because the counsellor will be unable to communicate much of what happens in a counselling interview because of its private and confidential nature. Furthermore the counsellor, like his clients, needs to express his doubts and feelings to someone outside the structure of the school. Supervising counselling casework is a highly specialized job and it is not one to be added to the burden of the head's duties. Yet we must face the fact that without regular discussion of the details of his counselling interviews with someone with the skills and the experience to help him, the counsellor's work may be stunted at best, damaging to others at worst. In other casework professions what social workers call 'supervision' is part of the job. But in so many areas there are neither resources available nor machinery yet operative for a counsellor's work to be thoroughly supervised. This is a serious omission. The counsellor training courses attempt some follow up and provide some refresher courses: this too I regard as essential, but it is not enough. The counsellor on the job needs regular on-the-spot case discussion and supervision.

Before I go on to discuss possible mechanisms for providing this kind of 'quality control' I want to elaborate further the extent of the counsellor's need, in the interests of his clients, for the kind of critical support which a tutor or supervisor can provide. Despite rigorous selection and thorough training the counsellor's true suitability or otherwise for his work may not emerge until he is actually on the job. Unless there is someone to encourage, stimulate and stretch him in his work he may find that the job is too difficult for him. If he remains alone, isolated and unsupported, either he may hide his problems behind a mound of paper work or fact-finding missions or he may become so anxious and insecure about his work that its calibre suffers.

During counsellor training it is not all that difficult to accept intellectually and academically the concepts and precepts of the counselling literature. Counselling practice, tape-recorded and properly supervised is certainly, like teaching practice, better than no practice at all. But, as any trained teacher knows, the difference between the cushioned leisure of teaching practice and the cut and thrust of a full timetable is enormous. In the counselling situation the contrast is even greater, partly because the job is more emotionally demanding than teaching and partly because the job itself is ill defined and arouses ambiguity and ambivalence on all sides. When the counsellor actually begins the job he really comes up against the problems of his own limitations. He may find that his actual behaviour is quite different from the behaviour his academic self would prescribe; for example he knows the sort of question he should not ask but he asks it because he is feeling insecure.

Furthermore he may find himself a prey to strong feelings which may interfere with his professional competence: anger, jealousy, anxiety, self-doubts, hatred. He may become over-involved with one pupil, dependent on another; he may collude with one client, or he may be totally manipulated or deceived by another. It would be a very abnormal counsellor who did not succumb, at least in part, to these sorts of feelings and pressures. What is important is to recognize, not to deny, that these feelings exist, and to improve one's counselling techniques through coming to terms with them. For a counsellor to deny the emotional repercussions a counselling interview may cause within him may block any growth and development in his work and possibly indirectly in his client. To face and accept his limitations and to make the best of them, the counsellor needs help–systematic, structured and specific help.

The counsellor needs help particularly in his first probationary year at work. But it is important to note that the need for counselling supervision does not disappear as the counsellor becomes more experienced, though it will not be needed so much. Counsellors need to be supervised weekly, fortnightly or monthly, according to experience, by someone appointed for this specific purpose. Local authorities could arrange casework supervisions for groups of counsellors, for individual counsellors or for both; in some areas this is already done. There is bound to be debate as to whether this person should be employed as part of the psychological, welfare or education service, whether he should be a psychiatrist, educational psychologist or psychiatric social worker or a counsellor. No matter: what is important is that the counsellor's work should be supervised. In an area with very few counsellors this could be a part-time appointment; it could be undertaken–as indeed it is undertaken in some areas–by the staff of the child guidance clinics. To appoint supervisory personnel specifically for counsellors is not an extravagance but an essential. If counselling is worth doing, it is worth doing well; bad counselling may be worse than no counselling at all. All counsellors have potential for good or bad; without supervision they may do as much harm as good, which may not only be distressing to individuals, but also a waste of time and money.

Let me not exaggerate the counsellor's dilemma. Any counsellor who has survived the hazards of selection and training should be capable of coping with the difficulties of his new job. But I would challenge the assumption sometimes made by sympathetic teachers that counselling is all for the good. It depends on the counsellor. If he is supported and helped in his work and not just left to go it alone he is more likely to do useful work. However many failings the counsellor has–and we must not forget that he is bound to have many–his weaknesses can be minimized and his strengths maximized if he is given help and encouragement both from his colleagues in school and in the community and from his 'tutor'.

In our experiment we have had to make our own unofficial channels of support and supervision. To an extent we have used many social workers in this role. The system we have evolved of regular case discussion with the child guidance staff is a good beginning but it is not official and it is not enough. The purpose of these discussions is more to help the counsellors make appropriate referrals than to improve the counsellor's insight, though this often happens as a side effect. To discuss all our cases, the ones we are to keep as well as the ones we are to refer, would entail meeting more often. Most of our cases are not referred to anyone, yet we still need help in handling them.

We have been helped unofficially in several other ways; my colleague and I insisted on being in school on the same days despite the complications this made to timetabling, because we recognize how much we are able to help each other through discussion. Apart from this we have been helped by the Marriage Guidance Council and also by a psychiatric social worker who has undertaken regular supervisions on a voluntary basis for four years. Her experience of working with disturbed adolescents has helped greatly in clarifying our role *vis-à-vis* the specialist services. Her unfailing concern and practical help have sustained me through many difficulties and without her I might long since have become faint-hearted and given up.

Apart from this help we have received as individuals we have also gathered together a group of counsellors working for our education authority. We have discovered some dozen counsellors of various kinds in our area; we meet about three times a term. Sometimes we discuss matters of role and organization, sometimes we discuss current cases or principles. We feel our self-help system has considerable value. We pool our dilemmas which eases the burden of them and makes us feel less isolated.

Selection of counsellors

The initial selection of teachers for counselling training is as important as the training itself if we are not to waste our resources training people who are not suitable for the job. The university courses are well aware of their responsibilities here. Their selection procedures stress the personality of the counsellor more than his academic qualifications; most courses demand a teaching qualification and five years' teaching experience, though in special circumstances those conditions can be waived. Some courses accept social workers but most are aimed at practising teachers.

The university counselling courses have developed their own criteria and techniques for selection which are constantly evaluated and reviewed. My additional plea is that, apart from a strictly supervised first year, counsellors should also be subject, like many businessmen, to an annual review of performance. It is essential, though certainly not easy, to keep high standards within the counselling profession. We must expect counsellors to make mistakes: that is why we need to provide tutors for counsellors. But any counsellor whose work continues to deteriorate in spite of supervision and support should be asked to give up counselling.

Training

On the difficult question of selection and training counsellors, I find myself much in agreement with Alick Holden. In chapter 5 of *Teachers as Counsellors* he advocates, as I would advocate, relatively short initial training courses with relatively little academic study and the emphasis on self-knowledge and counselling skills.[1] In both of us the influence of the Marriage Guidance Council must be acknowledged for it is just such methods of selection and training that are used by the Marriage Guidance Council. The courses in Education for Personal Relationships run by local education authorities, notably Gloucestershire and Wiltshire, use Marriage Guidance Council staff advisers but these are primarily courses for training teachers to lead discussions in personal relationships rather than for counselling, though of course one role often leads to the other. An adaptation and extension of this kind of scheme might well suit counsellors who want to specialize in personal counselling.

Such a scheme would not only provide the kind of help counsellors really need (ie in facing their own personal difficulties) but would also provide a more economical way of training counsellors and would make counselling a genuine option for a wider cross-section of the teaching community. To take these points in reverse order, we have to face the fact that some of the people most suited to be counsellors are not able for personal, usually family, reasons to go away for a year's training; indeed we might well question the desirability as a counsellor of someone who was prepared to leave his family for a year. This therefore rather limits the applicants—with exceptions no doubt—to unmarried men and women, or older men and women whose children are at least in their teens.

There is nothing amiss in this except that it makes it very difficult for the young married man (with at least five years' teaching experience) to go, and well-nigh impossible for a married woman, especially if she has children. Yet among these two categories there is I suspect much talent and enthusiasm for counselling. The married woman could be a particularly rich source of counselling talent. Part-time courses and regular supervision would suit both the local authority and the house-bound teacher, male or female. For the local authority they would make for great economies: the expense of seconding staff on full salaries for a year is great. For the individual teacher it would make it possible to work with emotionally deprived children without having to sacrifice one's own family in the process.

We need as counsellors people who lead balanced and integrated lives. Being married or having children is not an essential qualification for being a school counsellor; but it can provide relevant experience.

If we argue that counsellors should be teachers we might just as well argue that counsellors should be parents. The argument that counsellors should have taught rests on the following case: experience as a teacher helps the counsellor to be accepted by other teachers, to understand their point of view and to know what children are like in normal circumstances. It seems to me that the same case could be argued for experience as a parent. In my view these qualifications are desirable rather than essential. However if we want to attract younger people into counselling, we must provide more flexible training arrangements. The course at the Tavistock Institute of Human Relations, London, provides just this: one long evening a week for a year for teachers who wish to improve their counselling skills. They may become counsellors or they may remain teachers with special interest in their role as house master or form tutor. But the course is necessarily not overloaded with academic material and provides ample opportunity for supervised group discussion of on-going problems.

There is I think a distinction to be made between the full-time and the part-time counselling courses. The advanced diplomas in education with special reference to guidance and counselling provide an excellent general training; many of the products of these courses take up posts of special responsibility, perhaps as deputy head, or senior master or mistress, or head of house. Their special training and knowledge must be invaluable in these posts. Others take up posts specializing in vocational guidance and testing or in personal guidance; others combine these functions. Certainly to train a teacher for any of these eventualities takes at least an academic year if not two.

But do *all* counsellors have to learn all this? General all-purpose counsellors or outstanding teachers who want to become heads or lecturers in education certainly need at least a one-year course to acquire a sound background knowledge of sociology, psychology and guidance techniques: indeed it is not surprising to hear the products of the one-year training courses complain of intellectual indigestion. But professional skills for pastoral care for those preferring the teacher/counsellor role or for those wishing to specialize in personal counselling or improve their skills as house masters or form tutors could probably be taught a different way. An academic course spread over several years of one evening a week (rather like an extramural university diploma) might provide a more digestible form of background knowledge. The casework discussion, in groups and individually, should be considered a part of the job. Vacation courses could provide more intensive experience in groups without demanding too much sacrifice on the part of the counsellor's family. Many teachers are keen to learn professional counselling skills; more flexible training arrangements–as indeed are provided already by some local education authorities–would encourage, not discourage, these particular individuals. Teacher training courses too should at least introduce students to counselling; if student teachers could choose to specialize in counselling and follow this up with several more years of part-time in-service training we might find ourselves a source of economically but highly trained specialists; in their late twenties these teachers might be mature and experienced enough to specialize as counsellors.

Many people question the basic assumption that school counsellors should be teachers. Certainly some social workers, particularly married women with young families, are willing and able to work as school counsellors. They would need some knowledge of the education system, possibly some teaching practice, but they would have the advantage of being already orientated towards counselling techniques. Teachers often suffer more than they realize from what the French call *déformation professionelle*–much of a teacher's life is spent telling people what to do, giving advice, expecting to be obeyed and maintaining the *status quo*. To be good counsellors teachers have to be sufficiently flexible to change these habits.

To use teachers rather than social workers as counsellors is probably more economical in terms of manpower. Counsellors can always combine their job with teaching if necessary or go back into teaching later; thus the teaching profession is ultimately enriched, not deprived, by the counselling profession. The social work professions cannot afford to have their workers 'poached' into schools. On the other hand married women who cannot find social work to fit in with their children's school holidays might be prepared to take up school counselling or school social work precisely because of the hours. This is a gain, work for women who otherwise might not work at all. This is a source of skilled, already trained help which we must not overlook.

The career structure for counsellors

How should the counsellor fit into the educational hierarchy? Is counselling a 'promotion' or does this risk making it simply a stepping-stone for the ambitious? Is counselling to be dubbed a refuge for those who cannot teach, a backwater for those who want a quiet life? Should counsellors go on for ever or should they go back into teaching after a certain number of years? It seems to me that if counsellor selection is rigorous and careful then the purely ambitious or the 'failed' teachers should be eliminated. Inevitably some of the people attracted into counselling will have the ability and the desire to take headships later, whilst others will be content to counsel as an end in itself; this divergence and diversity within the counselling profession seems to me both desirable and normal. Counsellors who want to go back into the mainstream of teaching may enrich the teaching profession. Counsellors who want to counsel for ever should perhaps be asked to teach from time to time and their work should be evaluated. But they certainly should not be stopped from counselling if this is where their real talent lies.

In many schools counsellors are given posts of responsibility: this seems justifiable for the work is extremely responsible. Furthermore though respect from teaching colleagues should not depend on the size of one's responsibility allowance there is no doubt that it helps the acceptance of the counsellor if he has both on paper and in practice the status of a senior member of the staff.

Educational priorities

Introducing counselling into this country on any scale is expensive. When there is so little money available for expansion of the *basic* education services it is hardly surprising that education authorities are being cautious in appointing counsellors. The government and the Department of Education and Science, while following developments in counselling, have not committed themselves to it. The Seebohm Report came out against school counselling in favour of school social workers.

If we introduce counselling into this country on a large and systematic scale, then something else will have to go. If it came to a choice would we put counselling before the provision of nursery schooling for all or the reduction of size of classes in primary schools? If nursery and primary school facilities improved and if teachers generally knew more about counselling and social welfare would the need for counselling disappear? These questions are certainly impossible to answer until the effects of introducing counselling into schools have been evaluated. It would certainly be rash to launch into a wholesale counselling system for comprehensive schools without serious evaluative research on the subject, which also considered alternative solutions to serve the children's needs.

If we do introduce counselling into secondary schools on a large scale we must recognize that it will be an expensive process. First there are the costs of secondment, training and replacement. Then there is the decision whether to employ a counsellor instead of an extra teacher. There is the fact to be faced that whilst the teacher may teach a large number of children the counsellor will only help relatively few in depth in one year. It may well be far more important to give help in depth to a selected few rather than a little extra teaching to all. This is the same dilemma as we have in the social services, where the emphasis is switching to helping those who need help rather than providing blanket welfare benefits for all. But somewhere along the line these decisions about priorities have to be made. It is to be hoped that the decision about counselling will be based upon a rational evaluation of its usefulness. There may well be other more efficient and effective ways of helping adolescents at risk. Those of us who are enthusiastic about counselling must not forget this.

In their compelling and persuasive book, *Children in Distress*, Sir Alec Clegg and Barbara Megson demonstrate the need for more preventive work with children with problems. They argue that only about two per cent of our children are sufficiently badly behaved or disturbed to merit the help of the social services. They estimate that a further 10 to 12 per cent need preventive help and receive very little. They argue for a school counsellor who has a compassionate but unsentimental concern for the needs of children who have to cope with grave personal difficulties. They think as I do that this is a full-time job for one person; they estimate as I have found in practice that one in 10 children—that is, three in a form of 30—needs preventive help.[2] I too am convinced of the need but I am also concerned that the children's needs should be *met* and not overlooked in a flurry of activity in which organization takes over from counselling. Counselling is a response to an emotional need. We must start with the children's needs and organize our schemes to fit in with them, not the other way round.

References

1. A. Holden *Teachers as Counsellors* (Constable 1969)
2. A. Clegg and B. Megson *Children in Distress* (Penguin 1968)

Chapter 11

The counsellor as educator

In 1971 I changed jobs. I became deputy head of another comprehensive school. My belief in the value of pupil counselling remained unchanged, but I recognized more and more the need for similar work to be done with parents, staff, community and syllabus. My conviction was, and is, that counselling, far from being a frill, is an integral part of the education process. The more this unity is recognized, the more effective will be the education we provide. The pastoral care system of a school is not separate from the organization and curriculum, but is expressed through it. There is little point in adding a counsellor to a school where the pastoral care system is poorly conceived and barely executed; it is no good devising a brilliant pastoral care system if this in itself is separate from and contradictory to the academic system. In education, we need to spend time looking at the *total* message conveyed by the institutions we create. If we do this, we will find that the basic principles underlying both the counselling and the educational process are very similar. If they are not, then we may well have problems.

In recent years, the importance of good 'pastoral care' has been increasingly recognized.[1] So far so good. But in some cases, the unfortunate corollary of this welcome development has been for 'pastoral care' to be tacked on to a system, rather than integrated with it. Delegation of responsibility to a senior member of staff seems a wise step: but how often does delegation become relegation? Unless there is unity between the teaching and caring aspects of a school, as expressed through the organization, then there may result an unhealthy 'splitting', rather as children sometimes split parents into the 'kind loving' one and the 'harsh rejecting' one. In this situation, not only is there the risk of children playing one side off against the other. One section of adults may, wittingly or no, undermine what the other section is about, with resulting confusion and deadlock. Elizabeth Richardson's work[2] analyses this split in terms of task/sentient groups. She makes the point most emphatically.

It is vital that the same principles of pastoral care permeate the whole system, not be regarded as some kind of 'extra' to please those teachers who like to play at nymphs and shepherds. 'Caring' will of course include setting limits, and not allowing pupils to do as they like when they like, but the motive will not be to control, or to make the school easier for the administrators to run. Rather the aim will be to provide sufficient security to stimulate growth. Pupils need structure but not stricture. They will soon tell you the difference.

Unless the academic and pastoral are integrated there is a risk that the system itself will negate, undo, confuse or make impossible the work of the 'pastoral care' department. By the system, I mean not simply the overall organization, but also the timetable, the syllabus and the approaches to learning. There is for example no greater dictator of pupils' or teachers' lives than the timetable. The timetable can *prevent* form teachers being with their forms; they can *create* instability by moving pupils and staff round all the time; they can order our lives to the point where we can no longer exercise initiative. *Il faut manger pour vivre et non pas vivre pour manger.* The system is not there to make life easier for *itself*, but to serve the objectives of the school.

Underlying this discussion are several important counselling concepts, concepts which are in my view equally important to education: genuineness, trust and congruence. It is too easy in education to ignore the emotional implications of our intellectual decisions. In teaching we often fail to realize how many 'non-verbal' messages our institution will convey to its users. Nor do we always realize to what extent our users may be sensitive to contradictions between our stated objectives and what actually happens. For example a school may claim to like and respect its pupils, to value them, to wish to encourage their full development. Yet the organization of the school may spell out mistrust, the curriculum may stifle any active learning or any real growth and development in the individual, the relationships between staff and pupils may be based on fear or indifference, rather than love or commitment. We trust you; but we lock the doors between lessons. We value you; but we can't allow you to do anything for yourself in case you get it wrong. We want to prepare you for an adult role; in the meantime you must do as we say when we say it. We welcome parents; but only by appointment and preferably at our command.

This kind of *double entendre*, exaggerated as it may seem, is more common than most of us would admit. If the 'hidden curriculum' of the school belies its stated objectives, then the institution may appear not to be genuine. It may be difficult for pupils or parents to trust something which contradicts itself, yet trust is as fundamental to the learning process as it is to the counselling process.

If the discrepancy grows too great between what a school *thinks* it is doing for the pupils, what the pupils *feel* the school is doing, and what the pupils' actual needs are, then we have another counselling and educational malfunction: incongruence. If the administration is out of touch with the way pupils and their parents see the school, then misunderstanding and stalemate may ensue. In other words, for a school to function effectively there needs to be a large area of *congruence between pupils, parents, staff and community*.

Counselling and teaching

If we turn now to the teaching relationship itself, we find that at an expressive level, the basic requirements of an effective teaching relationship and an effective counselling relationship are one and the same: respect for each other, acceptance, trust, empathy, genuineness, non-possessive warmth and congruence. When we teach, we inevitably communicate our feelings about that class to the pupils, and vice versa. Any experienced teacher will know that if he is fed up with a certain class on a certain day, that class will immediately pick up these negative feelings and react accordingly. If we are frightened, our pupils become frightening; if we despise our pupils they become despicable; if we are not sure what we want from the lesson, our pupils will be confused and confusing; if we mean what we say, our pupils will take us seriously. In both a counselling and a teaching relationship (and indeed in relationships with colleagues and friends) we will inevitably communicate at a non-verbal level what we feel, whatever we say. Whatever their IQs, our pupils are not fools, neither are they easily fooled. If our message is false, then little learning will take place. Our pupils will not learn much unless there is trust between us, mutual respect, genuine caring, which will include not allowing ourselves to be duped, manipulated or unduly baited. In both teaching and counselling these are important factors.

Similarly the counselling process, which puts its emphasis on enabling an individual to face his own conflicts and problems for *himself* and to grow through them, is at one with the kind of teaching process where the pupil is enabled to learn for himself. Indeed, the trends in curriculum development and teaching methods which burgeoned in the early 70s seem more and more to confirm this unity. There is a growing tendency for 'personal development' to be included, either explicitly or implicitly in the curriculum.[3] Humanities projects, moral education, careers lessons, integrated studies, community education, thinking lessons, these all put the emphasis on helping the individual learn for himself.

They seek to give experience in taking responsibility for one's own actions, in making decisions; they aim to help individuals realize their potential and value their own experience and judgement. They should help to make pupils more self-aware, more confident, more sensitive to the needs of others, more able to choose a job when the time comes. As a result of these methods our pupils should be more articulate and questioning, active pursuers of learning rather than passive receivers of knowledge. For counselling and for teaching, the objectives are very similar indeed.

Counsellors and teachers

There are some tangible gains for teaching in schools where there are counsellors. Denis Lawrence's book[4] shows that in his school pupils who were counselled made substantially greater advances in reading than those who were not. Teachers have become more interested in the use of the small group as a teaching unit, particularly in mixed ability teaching.[5] In this the counsellor has experience and expertise to share, though it is vital that he himself can distinguish between group teaching, group discussion and group counselling.[6] It is inappropriate for a counsellor to indulge in some technique which he may have found beneficial in training but which may be inappropriate in the classroom situation.[7]

At all times the counsellor offers to the teacher a 'model' of behaviour: this in the sense of 'example' rather than perfect example. From this the teacher will learn indirectly, even unconsciously. In an article in *Trends in Education*[8] I have described in detail the kind of support and training a counsellor can provide for the teacher, making the significant point that the process is reciprocal and the counsellor will also learn from and be supported by the teacher.

Once a counsellor has established a position of being accepted and respected in the staffroom, he can then fulfil a more specific training role, by acting as group leader or consultant to various kinds of staff group, eg year or house teams, integrated studies teams, probationer staff or staff who are interested in developing further their counselling skills. None of this will work however unless the staff want his active support and unless he can define realistically what each group can and cannot do. He may be able to share with staff (and they with him) skills in interviewing, in writing letters to parents, writing reports for social workers, though most of what he teaches will be through practice rather than theory.

Like Leona Tyler,[9] I define a counsellor as someone who spends his time counselling! It may be difficult for a counsellor to spend a major part of his time on in-service training of staff, but there will be by now many ex-counsellors taking a senior teacher role with a large training element. Such a person may fulfil an important role in helping staff work through their feelings about policy developments and innovations. Elizabeth Richardson's work[2] has highlighted the importance of the dynamics within and between staff groups in the implementation of policy decisions.

The welfare team

There are many ways in which a counsellor's work can develop. Is he to concentrate on counselling pupils, or group work with pupils, work with parents, or family casework, work with staff, work with other agencies, or work with the environment of learning? In an article on community schools[10] I made the point that 'In the community school, whilst we need maximum contact and co-operation between the various workers serving that school, and a shared philosophy, we still need specialists and specialist skills. It is unrealistic for every worker to do everything. It is important to build a team.' Within the school the team must include a senior member of staff if the work is to remain integrated with the work of the school as a whole. In the second part of this chapter I shall describe how I took on such a role, as deputy head, no longer counselling but working with the environment of learning and leading a team which included a counsellor and a social worker.

Before doing this I want simply to make two more points about the counsellor. First I do not believe that the counsellor should be a change-agent in the sense of political activist; if he wants to change the school system, he should change his role, as I did. I was glad to hear Professor Halmos make the same point at an international conference of counsellors.[11] If as a result of counselling our clients decide to change the world, then that is their decision. Certainly this should not be the result of counsellor pressure, however subtle. In my view, the same applies to teachers.

The second point concerns the support and supervision of the counsellor. Too many counsellors are still left in splendid isolation to sink or swim. In 1971[12] I proposed that LEAs should establish systematic supervision of all counsellors, if necessary using existing educational psychologists, to safeguard and help both pupils and counsellor. There are still LEAs where there are too few official checks and supports for the counsellor in action.

Authority, role diffusion and boundaries: some dangers

Counselling and teaching methods are much intertwined: so in teaching the terms of 'non-directive', 'non-authoritarian', 'child-centred' are much in vogue, and sometimes used inappropriately. The skill in teaching and counselling is knowing *when* and *how* to be *what*! These concepts *rigidly* applied can make a nonsense, and more so in teaching than in counselling. A completely non-directive approach in the classroom can leave pupils totally baffled. A teacher has authority whether he likes it or not: he does not have to use it in an authoritarian fashion; when he has it but does not recognize it or use it, he leaves his pupils in the air. A teacher also has expertise, experience and knowledge: yet he appears at times to try to do anything but actually teach. He is a friend, social worker, confidant, enabler, facilitator, but not a teacher. Do our children really feel so put down if we put our knowledge and experience at their disposal? Do they really want our roles to be so blurred and confused? Ethel Venables's study of teachers and youth workers shows this is not so.[13]

Further there has come into play what I call the 'law of diminishing expectations'—'He can't help it, he's only a child', 'It isn't her fault, her family's got problems', 'Officer Krupke I'm really a slob' as the song in *West Side Story* puts it. This I see as a way of handicapping further the have nots, for he who expecteth nothing shall not be disappointed. Children are adept at playing up their weaknesses. Rewarded for this skill they only become weaker.

There is considerable evidence that young people thrive neither in authoritarian nor in *laissez-faire* climates.[14] Neither *extreme* is helpful to their development. To achieve a genuinely responsible atmosphere in which young people may grow, adults must neither dictate, nor simply leave young people to get on with it. They must provide support and an adult model which can be accepted, modified or rejected as appropriate. Adults cannot do this if they themselves are pretending to be adolescents. John Bazalgette sums this up very clearly in the conclusion to his book *Freedom, Authority and the Young Adult.*[15]

By 1972 I was sufficiently disturbed by this lack of adult leadership to add a note of warning. 'Some of the most distressed girls I saw as counsellor were those whose parents or teachers set no limits at all.'[16] For the adolescent in search of an identity, this kind of freedom can be paralysing, paralysing because the adolescent cannot grow in such insecurity, only search wildly for someone to show concern, for someone to assert an adult identity against which they can measure themselves.

The net result of this 'permissiveness' in adults was to push anyone in a counselling role into a position where they were under pressure to do what other adults were failing to do. This I regarded as a curious and undesirable role reversal. I am not saying that the counsellor should never set limits: he will do so, consciously and unconsciously, simply by his adult presence. But he cannot function if this becomes his main responsibility, for this is not his prime task. In 1971 I summarized the kinds of problems current at that time.[8] I found more and more that my role was to help individuals express the terrifying 'freedom' they were exercising, and to help them get sufficient confidence to tell their parents how they felt. It amazed me that so many parents failed to see what was happening under their eyes. I could only assume that they really didn't want to know, partly because they didn't know what to do.

Theory into practice

Much of what I have said so far is reflected in the work I went on to do as deputy head. In my new position, I quickly discovered what I had already suspected, that I could not effectively combine the roles of deputy head and counsellor, though there was inevitably a counselling component in my work. In this I differ from Alick

Holden[17] who claims to combine successfully the roles of deputy head, counsellor and teacher. My job as deputy head was not to do the counselling, but to see that it was done; to support those who were doing it; to ensure as great a harmony as possible between the academic and the pastoral. My principal clients were the staff, not the pupils or their parents. My methods had to be more direct, even directive. My skills were still there (and very useful in interviewing) but I had no unpressurized time at my disposal. The only individual pupils I attempted to counsel were those referred to me by counselling staff, usually at a remedial rather than a preventive stage. In other words, I was a prey to the usual pressures which beset a teaching member of the hierarchy: pressures of role, of time, and of organization.

Integration of pastoral and academic

Fortunately the head and staff had already perceived the need for integration of academic and pastoral: this is reflected through a timetable which favours block timetabling, and the teaching of most children in their own form rooms and in form groups. It is particularly reflected in the integrated studies programme for the first and second years, and the community education programme for the fourth years. The teachers themselves are well supported through the team teaching methods used.

Through integrated studies, the first and second year teachers spend two and a half days a week teaching their own forms, thus ensuring continuity of care, security of tenure and stability of relationships. Contact with parents is particularly encouraged through report days: reports are not sent home but handed over personally and discussed by form teachers, who are able to talk confidently both about academic progress and personal development. The teaching methods used are designed to encourage initiative, decision-making, and the taking of responsibility by individual pupils. The community education programme, a whole morning a week for all fourth years, is designed specifically to help prepare the pupils for their adult role. None of these innovations is easy to put into practice: indeed a school based training programme to evaluate the integrated studies teaching has been set up. But the fundamental philosophy recognizes the link between the form teacher's pastoral and academic role, a link which primary schools have long since fully exploited.

Preventive work in lower school

The counselling/welfare team itself was built up over a period of three and a half years. It began with the appointment of a teacher/social worker in lower school. Her job was divided into three parts:

to teach, to work with parents and to support staff, particularly heads of year. Her brief did not include counselling as such. The pupils in this school, and their parents, need a great deal of practical help and encouragement. The counselling orientation was there, but the approach was largely action orientated, bridging the gap between home and school, between home, school and social welfare agencies, reinforcing and encouraging attendance, pressing, where necessary and when parents wished, for financial help or even rehousing. Until these practical fundamentals were dealt with, counselling for these particular pupils seemed inappropriate, particularly since on the whole they are pupils who act out rather than internalize their problems.

Our next step was to undertake systematic screening of the first year intake, with a group reading/comprehension test, a maths test, a non-verbal reasoning test and finally a social adjustment scale filled in by the form teacher. The tests were done towards the end of the first term, after the children had settled in. The aim was to help us ascertain which individuals needed extra help and of what kind. The most valuable part of the testing programme was not so much the actual statistical scores (though occasionally interesting discrepancies of score and opinion arose) as the discussion between the form teacher, the social worker and myself which, though ostensibly about the pupil, did a great deal to develop and encourage the staff concerned. It also helped to counteract the crude labelling and stereotyping which might have come from a study of figures without facts. The next move was to decide upon strategies for helping each child in need. Not every child who appeared from these tests to be 'at risk' could be referred to the child guidance clinic nor did they need to be. But their all-round progress was carefully watched by the form teacher. Those children categorized as 'antisocial' rather than neurotic often responded well to firmer handling. Our educational psychologist was always ready to discuss individuals and advise on action where appropriate.

Alternative provision in lower school

After we did this research (and probably before it!) it was clear that there were some children who needed more help in the teaching situation than could be offered by the mixed ability form unit. Remedial teaching was already done by withdrawal of small groups (*not* by having a remedial stream). But some of the children's problems were not remedial so much as behavioural and psychological. A few of these children already went out of school for 'tutorial' classes, on certain sessions each week. We decided to start our own school based tutorial unit as well, hoping thus that it would be easier to keep pupils integrated with the main stream; and that we should thereby help more of the children needing special help. It took a long time for the staff as a whole to agree that this was needed and even longer to find the right teacher, capable of drawing up a frame of reference.

Included in our thinking was the concept of the 'nurture group' which was an idea developed in primary schools at that time. The theory was that some children needed 'nurturing' before they were ready to begin learning effectively; this nurturing would include feeding, playing with sand and water, learning, through adults, internal controls and strategies for coping. Many of the children at the secondary stage were as much in need of this fundamental 'family group' experience. The aim of the unit was not to separate the child from his peers, but rather to help him to integrate better with them and to benefit from the education provided. There were 10 sessions a week with children attending for a minimum of two sessions and a maximum of five. Entry and exit procedures had to be carefully monitored. But the unit (fundamentally a 'teaching' unit) did something which was *not* counselling yet which was more appropriate to the needs of those children.

The appointment of counsellors

The success of the teacher/social worker in lower school eventually created a demand for a similar worker in upper school. We were well served by the social services and had an education welfare officer who worked exclusively for our school. Nevertheless we found having our own worker so beneficial, specially in terms of work with parents, that staff were unanimous in creating yet another scale post from the teaching quota. For upper school, we deliberately chose someone more counselling-orientated, who was also capable of undertaking family casework and careers guidance where appropriate. Shortly after her arrival we also found a part-time counsellor for lower school, since by this time staff accepted the need for counselling as well as all the other provision. She works mainly with third years on the model I had used previously.

Next there came in upper school a demand for another special unit. This we called a 'compensatory unit', or C group, but its function was mainly to provide a home base for children who could not cope with the more academic rigours of upper school. All pupils were encouraged to attend their options, but some frankly could not cope with them, and needed a secure base from which to set off when they felt stronger. Truants returning, particularly those who were school phobic, also found this group a welcoming place to gain confidence to return fully. Disruptive and unmanageable pupils seemed to divide into two types—those who behaved badly because they could not do the work, and those who just behaved badly. Only the first kind were given refuge. The others were dealt with in the usual manner, though it would be fair to say that they still remain a problem to be worked at.

The welfare team

By the time the special unit was set up in upper school, the welfare department had grown enormously, with myself acting in effect as head of department. The link with the remedial department was very close. By then we had two full-time teacher/social workers, one part-time counsellor, one teacher in charge of the tutorial unit (lower school) and one in charge of the compensatory unit upper school. All of us worked closely with heads of years, their deputies and form teachers, also with the educational psychologist, education welfare officer and social workers in our area.

Group work for staff: in-service training

Our sense of identity was greatly increased by another notable development. Through links we already had with a nearby psychiatric teaching hospital, we were able to establish a monthly 'group discussion' for staff. This group went on for some two years, meeting each month. The dividend was not obvious immediately, but gradually we realized that, though the group itself did not take any action, we were able to ventilate our feelings in the group, to begin to say what we really thought, to trust each other because we were more honest with each other, and to take action outside the group.

The group was always 'open'. Initially a wide range of staff came, including some heads of years. Gradually the group consolidated into simply those staff directly concerned with social welfare, counselling and remedial work. Although it was not our original purpose to form a group for these particular staff, it was nevertheless just what we needed to supplement our more action-orientated departmental meetings.

We had foreseen the original purpose of the group as being to work on the school environment of the child. We were working on the theory that it was not enough to counsel the child, or the child and his parents. We had to look hard too at what the school was doing. We had no doubt that schools exacerbate, consciously or unconsciously, many of the problems about which they complain so loudly. We did not imagine that our school would be any exception. Some of these problems come from organization, some from curriculum, some from the kind of corporate ethos which grows up in a school, some from staff's own particular personality problems; all this apart from what the child is like. In any school, all these aspects need looking at, however painful the process may be. Our group did not purport to do away with the problems miraculously, but it did increase our understanding of them. Sometimes organizational changes could be made, sometimes we realized that our fears were just fantasies, feeding on our own insecurities.

We could not have run this group ourselves. I was a participant member. The group was led by a psychiatrist, who brought with him a psychiatric social worker, a clinical psychologist (all from the children's department of our nearest hospital), together with our own educational psychologist.

Support from the psychiatric services

Through our increasing link with the hospital we not only took part in various pieces of research, thus getting additional preventive help for our pupils, but also got support for our counselling staff, a 'hot line' for emergency cases. A further development is a weekly group for adolescents held in upper school, and run jointly by a psychiatrist from the hospital and our teacher/social worker. For some time we had the idea of establishing a group for deviants or for phobics. Neither came to fruition since the deviants deviated and the phobics never came! This group was carefully selected to make a balance between extroverts/introverts, conformists/non-conformists, fearless/fearful. From all accounts it has gone very explosively and certainly needed the expertise of the psychiatrist. It will be interesting eventually to try to evaluate the effect on group members and their effect on their peers.

The in-service training role of the deputy head

It is clear from what I have said that much of my time as deputy was taken up in supporting the developments I have so far described. But my brief as deputy was not simply to be 'head of guidance and welfare'; apart from the usual administrative and teaching duties which befall a deputy, I also had specific responsibility for students and probationers. In this role I used my experience as a counsellor as much as my experience as a teacher.

Students and probationers

For students I ran a weekly discussion group and gave occasional individual help to supplement the work of heads of department if necessary. Social work or counselling students had a regular individual supervision period either from myself or one of the teacher/social workers. I wondered whether *non*-social work students receive generally as much support? In many cases we do not make time for this in school, yet teaching students need as much if not more help.

For probationers I ran a special induction programme, which lasted three days and was followed by regular fortnightly working lunch hour meetings. I was an official probationer tutor for the area I served which meant I could offer further courses through the nearby teachers' centre. These included 'role play' and invaluable visits to primary schools. I often felt in individual discussion with probationers that they were reluctant to reveal their difficulties to me—the 'judgemental' role of the deputy was not to be escaped. Because of this, I appointed the next year a more junior member of staff to act as a less formidable father confessor. But his job was impossible for a different reason, not so much role, but time. In other words, looking after probationers is a *proper* job and needs time allocated to it. It must be added that on the whole staff, like adolescents, get a great deal of help from their own peer group and not from the person officially labelled 'probationer tutor' or 'counsellor'. But this does not mean that there is no need for either of the latter! My own support as a probationer tutor came from the monthly lunch with the other tutors in the area, most of whom were primary head teachers. Not only was I sustained by this group but I was able to start a two-way process of communication between our school and the primary school feeding it. This process was ostensibly at a factual level but in fact was to do with the building of trust, mutual respect and genuine co-operation.

Links with nearby schools

I was fortunate in having an existing link with yet another group of primary heads in the area. Within this group we planned and executed various in-service training activities, including two residential weekends. The intermingling of staff from various schools was always productive. But the most interesting of the activities we undertook was a further weekend run on our behalf by the Grubb Institute. Our aim was to study 'schools in their communities'. Seven schools participated, two secondary and five primary. Each secondary school sent seven representatives and each primary five. To record what happened would take another book! But as a result of this weekend, the amount of genuine co-operation between neighbouring schools increased enormously. The staff group who attended became revitalized and saw much more clearly where best to put their energy. There was set up between ourselves and our nearest feeder junior and infants school a monthly working lunch. For each meeting a different topic was taken, such as reading, integrated studies, transition from primary to secondary. Apart from the heads and myself, different staff were invited each time, a maximum of two per school. The plan was that a network of interrelationships between schools would be built up between those staff most intimately concerned with each topic. We planned eventually to do the same kind of work with other neighbourhood schools. With our neighbouring secondary school, we began an exchange and sharing of staff and facilities which seem so obvious now, yet would never have happened without the shared experience of the weekend.

Counselling and administration

I have given here a straightforward, albeit much abridged, account of some of the ways in which I used my experience as counsellor in my role of deputy head. An article in the *British Journal of Guidance and Counselling*[18] shows an increasing trend for counsellors to get key administrative posts, so it is important to look at the possible outcome of this trend.

It is interesting to note that all the developments which took place while I was deputy head were the result of teamwork, consensus and co-operation. They came with staff agreement, sometimes in fact at their request. This in itself is a counselling approach to management. My aim was, as in counselling, to give staff sufficient support for them to activate and use their own resources; not to 'take over' the work myself but rather to build strength in others, and to build a team. It was a difficult role with few immediate satisfactions. Yet after three and a half years it began to fall into place. The welfare team emerged strong and confident; one social worker began to organize her own weekly working lunch, the other undertook student supervision and intensive group work. The staff as a whole no longer sniped surreptitiously at the 'fancy work' done by the new team members. Heads of year began to be less threatened by new personnel and vice versa. Each member of the team began to work more effectively, each fulfilling his specific role, but in harmony with the others.

Like any system, this one is far from perfect and will continue to develop and evolve according to changes in needs. There are some incipient dangers, notably that of beginning to function more like a social welfare agency than a school. The prime function of a school is to educate, not to take over the functions of other agencies; to get other agencies to do their job, not to take on all the failures of other agencies. The social welfare agencies in the school are there to *back up* the academic aims, to enable the pupils to benefit from the education provided. We include in the education provided the development of the total individual, but in doing this we must not neglect his academic development. We have had to draw firm boundaries. Our reputation in the neighbourhood for dealing miraculously with impossible children has meant that we are constantly asked to take children that no one else can, apparently, deal with. We do not believe this to be so, nor do we feel it healthy that we should do so. This is like being the counsellor who must take on everything himself. Our first duty is to the children we have, many of whom need more help than we can ever provide.

The message is clear. We must not expect to perform miracles, but we must never give up trying. The more clearly we understand the *limits* of the job we are supposed to be doing, the more we understand and work at the irrational as well as the rational aspects of our task, the more likely we are to succeed.

In this chapter I have talked as much about education as about counselling. I have not been trying to make too many claims for counselling. Understanding of counselling principles can enhance the educational work of the school but it is not a substitute for education. The best of our teachers will instinctively incorporate counselling principles into their teaching. The best of our counsellors will instinctively contribute to a particular kind of learning. Yet the two jobs are different. It is only by understanding in which ways they are the same and in which ways they are different that each will be able to do his job properly.

References

1. M. Marland *Pastoral Care* (Heinemann 1974)
2. E. Richardson *The Teacher, the School and the Task of Management* (Heinemann 1973)
3. For example, Schools Council: Integrated Studies Project
   You in the Seventies (ILEA)
   Living Decisions (BBC)
   P. McPhail *Moral Education*
   E. de Bono *CORT thinking lessons*
   Various exercises in decision-making (CRAC) eg:
   B. Hopson and P. Hough *Exercises in Personal and Career Development*
   W. Law *Decide for Yourself*
   A. Jones, J. Marsh and A.G. Watts *Male and Female* and *Living Decisions*
   The Life-style Series (Hobsons Press 1974, 1977)
4. D. Lawrence *Improved Reading through Counselling* (Ward Lock Educational 1973)
5. B. Kaye and I. Rogers *Group Work in Secondary Schools and the Training of Teachers in its Methods* (Oxford University Press 1968)
6. S. Thompson and J.H. Kahn *The Group Process as a Helping Technique* (Pergamon 1970)
7. A.J. Grainger *The Bullring: A Classroom Experiment in Moral Education* (Pergamon 1970)
8. A. Jones 'School Counselling' *Trends in Education* Department of Education and Science no 23 (July 1971)
9. L. Tyler *The Work of the Counselor* (Appleton Century Crofts 1961)
10. A. Jones 'The All-Purpose, All-Age Community School' *The Youth and Community Review* no 22 (Spring 1972)
11. P. Halmos 'Counselling and Political Change' Paper at the 6th International Round Table for the Advancement of Counselling (Cambridge April 1974)
12. A. Jones 'What do School Counsellors Need?' *Comprehensive Education* no 19 (August 1971)
13. E. Venables *Teachers and Youth Workers: A Study of their Roles* (Evans Methuen Educational 1971)
14. R.K. White and R. Lippitt *Autocracy and Democracy: An Experimental Inquiry* (Harper 1960)

15. J. Bazalgette *Freedom, Authority and the Young Adult* (Pitman 1971)
16. A. Jones 'The School Counsellor' (Home and School Council 1972)
17. A. Holden *Counselling in Secondary Schools (with special reference to authority and referral)* (Constable 1972)
18. G. Antonouris 'Subsequent Careers of Teachers Trained as Counsellors' *British Journal of Guidance and Counselling* vol 2 no 2 (July 1974)

Bibliography

Counselling in Britain: theory and practice

Counselling in Schools Schools Council working paper no 15 (HMSO 1967)

P. Daws et al *'Who Cares?' A Discussion of Counselling and Pastoral Care in Schools* (Council for Educational Advance 1970)

P. Daws, J. Rayner, R. Atherley, J. Fuller, D. Juniper 'The Counselling Function: A Symposium' *Educational Research* February 1967

J. Fuller 'School Counselling: A First Enquiry' *Educational Research* February 1967

J. Gill 'Counselling in Schools' *Trends in Education* April 1967

P. Halmos *The Faith of the Counsellors* (Constable 1965)

A. Holden *Counselling in Secondary Schools (with special reference to authority and referral)* (Constable 1972)

A. Holden *Teachers as Counsellors* (Constable 1969)

'Horizontal Notebook on Pupil Counselling in Great Britain' *The New Era* November 1967

P.M. Hughes *Guidance and Counselling in Schools: A Response to Change* (Pergamon 1971)

R. Jackson and D.F. Juniper *A Manual of Educational Guidance* (Holt, Rinehart and Winston 1971)

D. Lawrence *Improved Reading through Counselling* (Ward Lock Educational 1973)

H. Lytton 'Counselling and Psychology in Britain' *Bulletin of British Psychological Society* October 1969

H. Lytton and M. Craft *Guidance and Counselling in British Schools* 2nd ed (revised) (Edward Arnold 1974)

P. Milner *Counselling in Education* (Dent 1974)

B.M. Moore *Guidance in Comprehensive Schools: A Survey* (NFER 1971)

F. Palmer *Student Guidance* (Longmans 1965)

E. Venables *Counselling* (National Marriage Guidance Council 1971)

K. Williams *The School Counsellor* (Methuen 1973)

Working Party Report on Counselling Services in Schools (National Association for Mental Health 1969)

American theory

D.S. Arbuckle *Counseling: Philosophy, Theory and Practice* (Allyn and Bacon 1965)

A. Boy and J. Pine *Client-centered Counseling in the Secondary School* (Houghton Mifflin 1963)

S. Hamrin and B. Paulson *Counseling Adolescents* (Science Research Associates 1950)

J. Krumboltz (ed) *Revolution in Counseling* (Houghton Mifflin 1966)

J. Loughary *Counseling in Secondary Schools: A Frame of Reference* (Harper 1960)
H. Lytton *School Counselling and Counsellor Education in the US* (NFER 1968)
C. Rogers *Client-centered Therapy* (Houghton Mifflin 1951)
C. Rogers *On Becoming a Person* (Houghton Mifflin 1961)
B. Stefflre (ed) *Theories of Counseling* (McGraw-Hill 1965)
C. Truax and R. Carkhuff *Towards Effective Counseling and Psychotherapy: Training and Practice* (Aldine 1968)
L. Tyler *The Work of the Counselor* (Appleton Century Crofts 1961)
J. Warters *Techniques of Counseling* (McGraw-Hill 1964)

Further theories and techniques of counselling, casework and groupwork

F. Biestek S.J. *The Casework Relationship* (Allen and Unwin 1961)
M. Ferard and N. Hunnybun *The Caseworker's Use of Relationships* (Tavistock Press 1962)
J. Heywood *An Introduction to Teaching Casework Skills* (Routledge and Kegan Paul 1964)
B. Kaye and I. Rogers *Group Work in Secondary Schools and the Training of Teachers in its Methods* (Oxford University Press 1968)
J. Klein *The Study of Groups* (Routledge and Kegan Paul 1956)
M. Moran *Pastoral Counselling for the Deviant Girl* (Geoffrey Chapman 1968)
J. Rich *Interviewing Children and Adolescents* (Macmillan 1968)
E. Richardson *Group Study for Teachers* (Routledge and Kegan Paul 1967)
C. Rogers *Encounter Groups* (Penguin 1971)
W.M. Schutz *Joy: Expanding Human Awareness* (Penguin 1973)
W. Sprott *Human Groups* (Pelican 1958)
S. Thompson and J.H. Kahn *The Group Process as a Helping Technique* (Pergamon 1970)
N. Timms *Social Casework: Principles and Practice* (Routledge and Kegan Paul 1964)
J. Wallis *Counselling and Social Welfare* (Routledge and Kegan Paul 1960)
J. Wallis *Marriage Guidance: A New Introduction* (Routledge and Kegan Paul 1968)

Adolescence: theory and background

J. Bazalgette *Freedom, Authority and the Young Adult* (Pitman 1971)
B. Davies and A. Gibson *The Social Education of the Adolescent* (ULP 1967)
N. Dunn *Up the Junction* (MacGibbon and Kee 1963)
E. and M. Eppel *Adolescents and Morality* (Routledge and Kegan Paul 1966)
E. Erikson *Identity: Youth and Crisis* (Faber and Faber 1968)
T. Fyvel *The Insecure Offenders* (Chatto and Windus 1961)
G. Goetschius and M. Tash *Working with Unattached Youth* (Routledge and Kegan Paul 1967)
J. Hadfield *Childhood and Adolescence* (Penguin 1962)
C. Hamblett and J. Deverson *Generation X* (Tandem 1964)
J. Hemming *Problems of Adolescent Girls* (Heinemann 1967)
E. Hurlock *Adolescent Development* (McGraw-Hill 1951)
C. Jones-Davies and R.G. Cave (eds) *The Disruptive Pupil in the Secondary School* (Ward Lock Educational 1976)
I. Josselyn *The Adolescent and His World* (Family Service Association of America 1959)
D. Miller *The Age Between: Adolescents in a Disturbed Society* (Cornmarket Hutchinson 1970)
M. Morse *The Unattached* (Penguin 1965)
F. Musgrove *Youth and the Social Order* (Routledge and Kegan Paul 1964)

M.K. Pringle *The Needs of Children* (Hutchinson 1974)
M. Schofield *The Sexual Behaviour of Young People* (Longmans 1965)
W. Wall *Adolescents in School and Society* (NFER 1968)
R.K. White and R. Lippitt *Autocracy and Democracy: An Experimental Inquiry* (Harper 1960)

Books about personal relationships and sex for adolescents and parents

K. Barnes *15+ Facts of Life* Family Doctor Series (British Medical Association)
K. Barnes *He and She* (Penguin 1958)
Boys' Questions Answered (National Marriage Guidance Council)
R. Cave and D. Conochie *Living with Other People* (Ward Lock Educational 1965)
R. Cave and R. O'Malley *Education for Personal Responsibility* (Ward Lock Educational 1967)
D.M. Dallas *Sex Education in School and Society* (NFER 1972)
Girls' Questions Answered (National Marriage Guidance Council)
R. Hacker *The Opposite Sex* (Pan Piper 1961)
A. Harris *Questions About Living* (Hutchinson Educational 1968)
A. Harris *Questions About Sex* (Hutchinson Educational 1967)
A. Ingleby *Learning to Love* (Robert Hale 1964)
Is Chastity Out? (National Marriage Guidance Council)
R. Morton *VD and Diseases Transmitted Sexually* Family Doctor Series (British Medical Association)
R. Pilkington *Facts of Life for Parents* Family Doctor Series (British Medical Association)
G. Prince *Teenagers Today* Family Doctor Series (British Medical Association)
C. Rayner *A Parent's Guide to Sex Education* (Mini Corgi 1968)
L. Richards *Design for Living for Boys* (Basil Blackwell 1963)
M. Richards *Design for Living for Girls* (Basil Blackwell 1963)
Sex Education in Perspective (National Marriage Guidance Council)
B. Spock *Problems of Parents* (Bodley Head 1963)
P. Vaughan *Family Planning* (Queen Anne Press 1969)
Where on Drugs: A Parent's Handbook (Advisory Centre for Education)
A. Wood *Drug Dependence* (Corporation of Bristol and Bristol Council of Social Service)
Your Teenagers (National Marriage Guidance Council)

For the full booklist of the National Marriage Guidance Council write to Bookshop, The National Marriage Guidance Council, Rugby.

Social and psychological services for young people

M. Carter *Into Work* (Penguin 1967)
The Education of Maladjusted Children Department of Education and Science pamphlet no 47 (HMSO 1965)
Guide to the Social Services (Family Welfare Association)
J. Kahn *Unwillingly to School* (Pergamon Press 1964)
I. Maclean *Child Guidance and the School* (Methuen 1966)
Psychologists in Education Services the Summerfield Report (HMSO 1968)
Report of the Committee on Local Authority and Allied Personal Social Services the Seebohm Report (HMSO 1968)
Report of the Committee on Maladjusted Children the Underwood Report (HMSO 1956)
E. Venables *Teachers and Youth Workers: A Study of their Roles* (Evans Methuen Educational 1971)
P. Willmott *Consumer's Guide to the British Social Services* (Penguin 1967)
Youth and Community Work in the 70s (HMSO 1969)

General background

M. Argyle *The Psychology of Interpersonal Behaviour* (Penguin 1967)
E. Berne *Games People Play* (Deutsch 1966)
G. Carstairs *This Island Now* (Hogarth Press 1963)
Children and Their Primary Schools the Plowden Report (HMSO 1967)
A. Clegg and B. Megson *Children in Distress* (Penguin 1968)
M. Craft et al *Linking Home and School* (Longmans 1967)
J. Douglas *The Home and the School* (MacGibbon and Kee 1964)
15 to 18 the Crowther Report (HMSO 1959)
Half Our Future the Newsom Report (HMSO 1963)
Higher Education the Robbins Report (HMSO 1963)
S. Jackson *A Teacher's Guide to Tests and Testing* (Longmans 1967)
M. Marland *Pastoral Care* (Heinemann 1974)
M. Pringle *Investment in Children* (Longmans 1966)
E. Richardson *Authority and Organization in the Secondary School* (Macmillan Education 1975)
E. Richardson *The Teacher, the School and the Task of Management* (Heinemann 1973)
B. Wootten *Social Science and Social Pathology* (Allen and Unwin 1959)

Information about training for counselling

D.H. Hamblin and A.G. Watts *Training Courses for School Counsellors* (CRAC, Cambridge)

Counselling journals

British Journal of Guidance and Counselling (CRAC, Cambridge)
The Counsellor Journal of the National Association of Counsellors in Education

Associations concerned with counselling

National Association of Counsellors in Education (NACE)
Hon Sec: Mr Terry J. King, 'Compton', 120 Straight Road, Old Windsor, Berkshire, SL4 2FB

Association for Student Counselling
Chairman: Mr Brian Thorne, University of East Anglia, University Plain, Norwich NR4 7TJ

Standing Conference for the Advancement of Counselling
(An umbrella organization to co-ordinate counselling in this country)
Secretary: Mrs Joan Burnett, 26 Bedford Square, London WC1B 3HU

International Round Table for the Advancement of Counselling (IRTAC)
(This organization promotes international conferences on counselling)
Chairman: Mr Hans Hoxter, Centre for Studies in Counselling, NE London Polytechnic, Livingstone House, Livingstone Road, London E15

National Institute for Careers Education and Counselling (NICEC), Bateman Street, Cambridge